101

MASSAGE TIPS AND TRICKS FOR THE NEWLY QUALIFIED THERAPIST

WHAT I WISH I HAD KNOWN WHEN STARTING OUT!

D SOWDEN

First Edition: 2014

ISBN: 1495452212
ISBN-13: 978-1495452215

DEDICATION

I dedicate this book to my wonderful partner Steve who has had to endure all my massage practises over the years and constant 'massage talk'.

Also to the wonderful massage tutors who helped develop my skills and knowledge and build the foundations for my massage career.

CONTENTS

PERSONAL ETIQUETTE

How we look and dress reflects how we view our business and influences the way others perceive our practice.

1. Massage oils and your lovely locks!

How we look has a definite relation between how our business is perceived by others. If you don't keep yourself clean, tidy and presentable then it can lead to questions on whether your business and materials are clean, tidy and fit for use. Keeping hair clean and presentable can be difficult when you are often accidentally wiping oil in your hair! Greasy, oil filled hair is never a good look, even if it does mean your hair is being conditioned!

One way around this is the fantastic invention of dry hair shampoo, which can easily be bought at any supermarket or local beauty store. It works wonders at drying up the grease and allowing the hair to stay a little fresher for longer, especially when the cause of dirty looking hair is as a result of massage oil which tends to get everywhere! Keep your hair clean and tidy and your business looks clean and tidy too!

2. Keeping time!

When carrying out a treatment we need to consider how were going to time the treatment. Cutting short the treatment is going to leave your client very annoyed which is rather frustrating if you didn't mean to and had only done so by not knowing the time.

These days very few people have clocks hanging around their home, therefore your going to need your own means of telling the time. This could be done via your phone, however this comes across as unprofessional and you have to fiddle to get it out of your pocket or to wherever you have kept it, mid treatment. I can assure you I have done this in the past and it isn't much fun!

A far simpler, easier and professional way of making sure you never cut short the treatment is using a nurses watch pinned to your uniform. It's easy to check the time, quickly and without any fuss and continues to maintain that professional persona. These can be picked up easily either online or a local shop.

3. Tunic, T-shirt or what to wear.

What you wear is a personal preference and there is no set rule, perhaps only one, remain looking professional. That means no dirty T-shirt from a night out in the pub! Seriously, it is completely up to you, but naturally something that is not very revealing and something that is easy to move around in. Now is not the time for tight fitting jeans if you are having to move muscles and body parts around.

Equally what you wear is once again, an indication of you and how you perceive your business. Wearing something smart, whether it be a polo top with your logo on or a beauty tunic, all help to instil confidence in clients that you are a professional and know what you are doing. Ideally you need to be wearing something that is comfortable for you to move around in, is clean, smart and allows ease of movement. People often opt for a tunic or T-shirt with dark trousers or comfy three quarter lengths.

Image can be very important at conveying impressions and part of massage is instilling confidence in clients that you can help them. By wearing clothes that look professional and smart it reflects that you mean business, helping to reassure clients that you can help.

"At work, dressing well can clinch your exuberance for your career, showcase your exuberant qualities and secure your confidence."

Lindsey Shores. www.forbes.com

IMPORTANCE OF COMMUNICATION

If we don't communicate with clients how do we expect to know how they think or feel about our business and what they require from us.

4. Find a way to communicate with clients.

Sometimes a business is successful, not just because of how good you are, but because you have the skills to build rapport with your clients and make them feel heard and listened to. Think about how you would like to be treated or how you would chat with a friend and apply those principles when you are talking to clients. You want your client to feel at ease and you can do this by being friendly and approachable and making conversation with them.

5. Listen to what clients want.

There is no point asking a client where it hurts or what areas they want working on if you are only going to do your own thing. This may seem obvious but you would be surprised how many clients say they told their therapist what specific areas they wanted working on, only for the therapist to glaze over this area or not include it at all. If a client wants more time spent on their left shoulder, then do this or explain why your choosing not to focus on this area. Follow through on their specific requests. Make clients feel listened to and they are likely to keep coming back.

6. Explanations are important.

After the massage has finished I often explain to my clients what I have found during their treatment. This is to make them aware of how their body feels and what's going on within their body. It helps clients to understand their bodies further allowing them to develop a deeper body awareness. It helps clients to make connections between their body and mind enabling them to become more in tune with themselves. Clients can use this to become aware of when their body is experiencing restriction or tightness and realise what areas are problematic. Equally they can use it to understand what areas need further treatment such as through more specific exercise.

Many a time I have been massaging people who thought that the trapezius muscle on the tops of the shoulder, was bone as it was rock solid! Once I explained that it was in fact tension and muscles should not feel that hard they began to make some connections, along with feeling confident in my abilities to help them. By explaining to clients how the body has felt to you and what areas of restriction or tightness you have come across, this often instils confidence into clients that you have the expertise and skills to perform the treatment and help with their body issues.

7. Why we do what we do.

Again communication is important, without it clients can be left feeling bemused and a little confused, especially if during the treatment, time has been spent on other areas than expected. Another reason to explain what areas have felt tight and where tension was found, is in order to clarify matters and help clients to understand further.

A client may have told you the problem was on the left side of the back when in fact the issues actually stemmed from the right side and as such, time was spent loosening that area up so the left hand side of the back could become free. This often helps clarify matters for my clients, as one client said to me 'I did wonder why you were working the left side as I had been feeling the pain on the right side, but I understand now and it all definitely feels a lot better.'

8. Client feedback.

Getting feedback from clients is important as it allows you to find out how they felt about the treatment. This helps you ensure you provided the best possible treatment as it's all about helping clients and getting them to come back! It also gives them an opportunity to consider how they feel after the treatment and in particular the benefits and after effects so they can stop and consider how much looser they felt.

At the end of each treatment I ask my client 'How's it all feeling?' so that they can stop and consider how their body is. This is so they can tell me how the treatment was, such as if it felt very tight over the shoulder blade as we were working on it, this way we could look more in depth at that area next time. Once again, it makes clients feel valued, that you haven't just taken their money and run, but are interested in them, how they feel and are ensuring they got the best from their treatment.

TAKING CARE OF YOU

We can't take care of others if we don't take care of ourselves first.
Take care of your own needs so you can help others.

9. Hands aren't everything!

I lose count of the times that clients have asked me if my hands hurt at the end of a massage! The answer is no and I have been working as a massage therapist for six years now. The reason they don't hurt is that I realise hands aren't everything! I make full use of my elbows, forearms, knuckles and fists in order to deliver a treatment that can be deep or firm yet less pressure on myself.

10. Look after those hands!

One of the reasons massage therapists tend to use other parts of their body instead of just their hands is to protect their wrists and to continue being able to work. If you continue to just use your hands and fingers then you will notice repetitive strain injuries setting in. I have often seen it quoted that between two and three and a half years is the life span of a massage therapist particularly when they use their hands alone*. Hence if you want to make a career in this business you need to look at ways to prolong your hands!

*American massage therapy association statistics.

11. Use of forearms.

The introduction of other body parts can take some of the stress away from your hands, helping to prolong your massage career and obtain deeper pressure. The forearm is a long bone and the muscles can help to get a lovely long even stroke which is helpful at warming a client's muscles up and allows a firmer pressure to be applied. By using the forearm to warm the muscles deeper work can then begin with fists and knuckles, as well as more sustained pressure from the forearms themselves.

The forearm is particularly beneficial for areas such as the hamstrings, calves and back. It enables you to cover a wider surface area so that more of the body is being massaged and enables you to give a pressure that the hands alone could not give. They provide a break from using your hands so they become less fatigued and less susceptible to repetitive strain injury. Although it may feel a bit strange at first, mastering the use of your forearms can help save your hands and can give the kind of pressure your clients like.

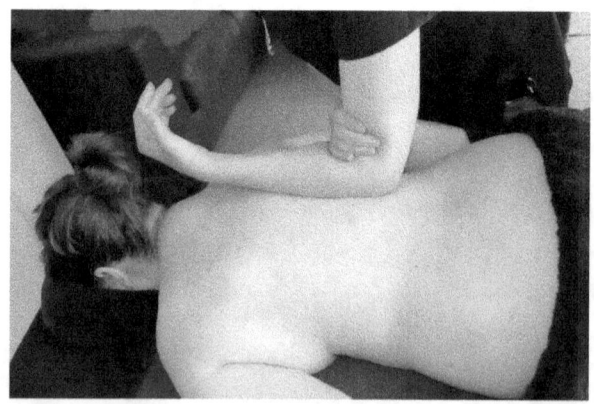

The best way to find out about using forearms, is to attend one of the many varieties of hands free workshops. There you will find out how to protect your hands as well as the best way to use forearms and other body parts. Body mechanics and using the body effectively is key to prolonging your massage career

12. Using knuckles and fists.

The knuckles and fists allow a great amount of pressure to be applied to the muscles with less impact on you, the therapist. By using a relaxed fist you can cover a large area with a deeper consistent approach. Always remember though not to tighten up the fist otherwise you will build up tension in the tendons of the hand.

The pressure from the fist allows you to sink deeper into the muscle, whereas the knuckles allow you to work more specifically into deeper knots and areas of tension and can be used for more specific work. Circular rotational movements can be used particularly on areas of the back such as the shoulder blades and tops of the shoulders, in order to help break down the tension. They help to protect your hands by allowing you to use various other body parts to carry out the treatment instead of relying solely on your hands. You can learn more about these techniques through advanced massage courses.

13. Keep your hands healthy.

Shortly after qualifying as a massage therapist I found out about a wonderful book created to help you look after your hands and their health. Written by massage student Lauriann Greene, who experienced pain in her wrists shortly after completing training. It lists various techniques to keep your hands in the best possible shape, from exercises to correct body posture. I would encourage you to look into this book so that you can delay the onset of any wrist issues and can find out further details on the sorts of exercises that help to look after your wrists and hands.

'Save your hands!: Injury prevention for massage therapists.'

Lauriann Greene

You can keep your hands healthy by learning techniques that involve using other body parts, stretching out your hands, keeping your hands relaxed and taking regular breaks.

14. Hand extension/flexion exercises.

Our hands are our most important asset when running a massage business and they need looking after well. Sadly, far too often they are overlooked and we only consider them when pain and issues arise. Try and get in to good habits now and be preventative when it comes to your hands. It's far easier to prevent issues before they arise instead of reacting to the tension and shortening of tendons in the hands.

A few helpful exercises are hand extension and flexion exercises. They are simple yet effective exercises which can be performed whilst you wait for your client to get ready before and after the treatment. Before starting the treatment it's advisable to get the body and hands warmed up, ready for them to be exercised through you performing massage. A great way to do this is to shake the hands repeatedly for around a minute until you can feel them nicely warming up. You can also do repeated big circles with your arms for thirty seconds to get your shoulders loosened up. These exercises are used in Chinese yoga and can be found freely on the internet. They are all simple techniques but help to get your body ready to carry out the treatment.

At the end of the massage and whenever you find yourself with a spare moment, you can do hand extension and flexion exercises. Hand extension exercises can be performed with you stood up, arms straight out in front of you at shoulder height with palms pointing upwards. Then with the other hand, gently and slowly stretch the hand backwards so you can feel a stretch in the front of the hand, into the wrist and the anterior forearm. Hold for ten seconds and repeat.

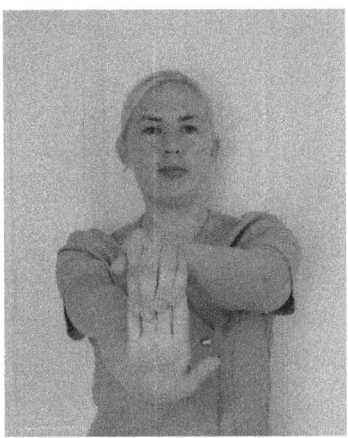

For the hand and wrist flexion exercises, you start in the same position, with the arm outstretched but this time with the elbow bent slightly and the palm pointing down. Then with the other hand you grasp the back of the fingers and hand and slightly and lightly pull the fingers back so the fingers point down as you straighten your arm due to the stretch placed on the wrist. This will give a stretch in the wrist and forearm. Then if you bend the fingers further back you will feel a stretch in the back of the hand and fingers. Hold for ten seconds for each part and then relax and repeat again.

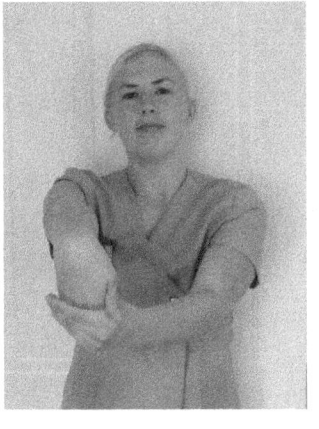

Our hands need looking after well and these simple exercises can be part of a balanced programme to take the best possible care of our most precious asset.

15. Hands free courses.

There are various reputable and credible courses out there designed to teach you methods and ways of massaging without using the hands, or at least less hand work. Having done a few courses in various no hands techniques I would recommend them as a way of maintaining and ensuring you stay healthy within your business practice. These courses look at ways that you can use the forearms, knuckles and fists, as well as how to support your wrist whilst working so it's not kept in a vulnerable state.

If you want to maintain a career in massage there a worthwhile investment. Aimed at helping to keep injuries at bay and include looking at issues of posture and the importance of keeping your body relaxed during massage. Learn these techniques now whilst you are starting out and you won't have the opportunity to build up bad habits!

16. Importance of relaxed body posture.

It can be easy when starting out to be so focused on the massage itself and ensuring your client loves their treatment, you forget to think about you and the need to protect yourself. How many of us heard whilst training, to relax our shoulders and that they weren't meant to be up around our ears?! Even since qualifying and continuing my professional development I have heard those words said to me!

It's important to have relaxed body posture when giving massage so that you don't build up tension in your own muscles. A relaxed body posture makes your body more fluid which then transpires into the massage, helping your massage to flow better and feel less rigid. Shoulders that are raised and hunched up are likely to result in a more restricted and inflexible massage as your not able to move as freely. If your body posture is not relaxed, then you are likely to build up tension within your body so that you now become the one with the achy back and problem shoulders. Next time you find your shoulders up around your ears, take a deep breath and drop them down, remembering to relax and let the massage flow!

17. Keeping hands relaxed.

It's easy in the beginning of your career, to be intensely focused upon the treatment and what your doing, that you end up working with very tight fists and hands. This can end up with the client experiencing a less than relaxed treatment as the hands and fists feel differently when clenched. It causes tension to build up in the fists and hands. The more relaxed the hands, the less tension that builds up, as you are no longer holding your fists so tightly that you would break something! It also means your hands are now relaxed and provides a greater feeling for the client.

So, when you find yourself holding your hand as stiff as as sword, remember to RELAX! If you find this difficult, then try shaking your hands to loosen them up! Allow yourself to relax into the massage and go with the rhythm and flow of the treatment.

18. Put your body weight into it!

Often people comment and wonder how I can put all that pressure into the massage and work so deeply when I am so little! The reason being, I have learnt that by putting my body weight into the massage I get a deeper treatment but with less effort required from me. It's simple to put your body weight into it by just leaning slightly over the table. By using a good body stance and ensuring the power does not come from the hands but comes from the rest of your body. You need your feet firmly on the ground so that you have correct balance and can apply an even weight down on your client.

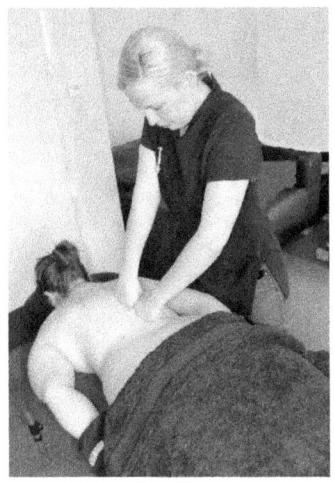

Equally you can stand with one leg behind the other with a mid to wide gap such as when you are doing a calf stretch. This way you can lean into the table and client and allow yourself to put your body weight into it.

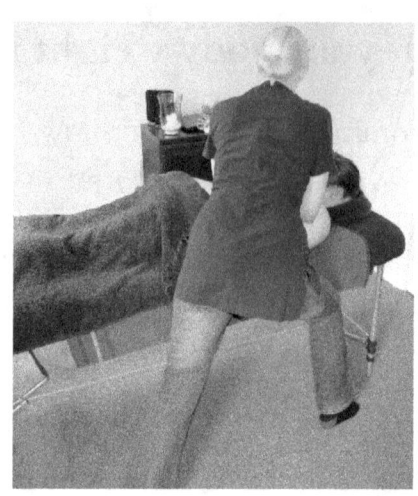

You'll know when you are using your full body weight as your likely to get less tired due to using your whole body, rather than just your hands and forearms. These techniques can be learned through advanced courses and no hands techniques.

19. Keeping your body healthy and strong.

In order to keep your business running and maintain your level of clients you need to make sure you look after yourself. You need to be keeping your body healthy so your not stood there massaging with an aching back envying your client! That means thinking about what you put into your system and how you treat your body. We all know more than five portions of fruit and veg a day are good for us but how many of us consume that many. If I told you that your business could rely on it, you might think differently! Watching what we put into ourselves helps to keep our bodies strong and healthy.

There are also a range of exercises that can help to strengthen the back and core muscles which will help with all the standing. Pilates and yoga have long been sited for their ability to strengthen the core muscles and back muscles which in turn help support the back and keep our bodies feeling supple.*
*HTTP://www.nhs.uk/Livewell/fitness/Pages/pilates.aspx
Strengthening our bodies now with regular exercise will be of benefit in the long run. Our bodies will learn to build up strength in key muscles used for massaging and to counteract problems from leaning over the table or from fatigued muscles.

When we exercise and eat right, it keeps our bodies healthy and helps boost the immune system so we're less prone to illnesses, resulting in less time off work.**http://www.firststeps-surrey.nhs.uk/healthy-eating-physical-activity/ Join the gym or create your own workout programme, but do something to get your body active and being treated well.

INNER INSTINCTS

Trust your instincts, and make judgements on what your heart tells you.

20. Listen to your inner self.

Clients often remark on how I 'just seemed to know the exact areas to work on' and their 'achy areas!' This comes through practice as your hands develop the sensitivity to peoples bodies and you get an idea of what your feeling for. However, I have had massages with people who have been practising for numerous years and sadly you can tell that they are working largely from what you've told them. Rather than listening to that inner voice that is saying *'I can feel some restriction, I think the shoulder's tight because the pectoral muscles at the front are tight'* they choose to follow a routine and won't deviate. They remember the routine they were taught at college and common solutions to typical areas and they carry these out, without using their initiative or instincts.

All bodies are different though and you need to become in tune with that specific client's body and listen to how your inner voice is telling you to work. Just because someone's issue doesn't follow the text book case or what you were taught in massage school does not mean that you shouldn't go with your gut instinct.

21. Gut instinct.

I know I have already mentioned this, but it has to be mentioned again due to it's importance! Listening to yourself and what your gut instinct is telling you about someone's body is vital. Not only in helping relieve any issues they may have, but when clients see that you are following your instincts, that you are effectively listening to their body and being in tune with them, they feel they are getting a fuller and more effective treatment and indeed they are.

Many of my clients have stayed on after problems have been fixed because they felt I had such a deep understanding and intuitiveness about their body that they felt it would be good maintenance for them. They have often commented on how 'It is so nice to receive a treatment where you just seem to know exactly what you are doing'.

MASSAGE TIPS AND TRICKS

Learn the tips and tricks to take your massage business from good to great.

22. It's all connected.

One major piece of advice, never forget how connected the body is. Remember that song from school about the bones and how the 'thigh bone is connected to the hip bone' that applies to the muscles too!* Muscles are all interconnected, hence when someone comes in and tells me they are having lower back pain, I'm thinking possibly tight glutes, tight hamstrings, even tight shoulders that could be affecting the body's alignment and structure and having a knock-on effect. Always remember how everything is connected, so when you are massaging one muscle you are massaging them all!

*James Weldon Johnson, Dem bones

23. Learn the body.

With the muscles and skeletal structure all being connected, you really need to know the body and be aware of the different muscle groups and consider their connections. For example, one of my clients came to me with a tight calf muscle from a previous tear to the achillies tendon, we began working on the hamstring, calf and achillies and although we had some relief it was still problematic.

I had chosen not to listen to my gut instincts because, if I'm honest I was a little intimidated by the client's previous therapist. However I decided that I needed to listen to my own thoughts and what I felt needed working on based on the remaining muscles and joint movement. That's when we began working on the calcaneus and rest of the foot and boy was that tight! After the first session working on the back of the leg and foot my client noticed an immediate difference.   Never be afraid to think outside the box and consider how the body is all connected.

Learning these connections can help you to develop a more proficient massage service, because instead of just looking at the issue you are looking at the whole picture or whole body! You can learn how one muscle or movement impacts upon another. Another great example of this is tightness in the shoulders. People often forget to consider the 'front shoulder' which includes the pectoral region. Seeing as so many people sit in front of computers, causing shortening of the pectoral muscles, it's very often the case that if you want the shoulders to release then you need to open up the chest first.

24. Tracing the body.

Learning the body goes hand in hand with tracing the body, feeling the muscle, the way it runs, the way it may pull over to one side more than the other, the way the shoulder blades may be too tightly together. These are all indicators for areas to work on and by tracing the body with your hands and fingers, seeing which way the muscles run, you get an idea of what needs working on.

You can feel the muscles with your fingers, the way some may be shortened or the impact that restricted muscles are having on the next muscle. An example of this is when the pectoral muscles in the chest are tight and they are pulling the shoulders round. You can trace with your fingers how the muscles feel, like their pulling round to the front, including how, when you get to the deltoid you almost want to scoop the muscle back. You may even find that whilst your tracing and following the muscle you come across other restrictions you hadn't anticipated, always follow it along and see what surprises come up!

25. Wibble wobble like jelly!

One of the best pieces of advice I was given was 'wibble wobble like jelly!' No, we're not going to be talking about yummy jelly here, but rather what we can do to stubborn muscles which refuse to loosen up enough for us to get in there and break them down. A solution, wibble wobble them like jelly!

Muscles such as the calf respond very well to this vibrational technique especially when their particularly tight as otherwise they can be very painful to work on. In order to get them to loosen up enough to be worked on, you can literally shake and wobble them as if you were shaking a bowl of jelly. You want to be creating a wibble wobble sensation in the muscle. The muscle finds this vibrational sensation confusing and doesn't know how to respond, so instead the brain tells the muscle to relax and they begin to let go of tension. The vibrational technique helps to free up restricted fibres and promote circulation.

It may sound bizarre, but the muscle responds by loosening up and relaxing. This means you suddenly have your way into the muscle and areas of restriction, releasing them further. This is best done lightly to begin with and then you can proceed to a slightly firmer pressure to get in to those particularly stubborn areas. You literally place your hand or hands on the client and begin to wibble and wobble. With regards to length of time, start with twenty seconds and see what the result are, you can always come in with a bit of massage and then apply some more vibrations and wobbling to the muscle and increase the pressure of the movement.

I learnt about this technique after struggling with a client who regularly had tight calves and always found them painful. Feeling perplexed, I asked a tutor on a course I was attending for tips on how to loosen tight calves. They informed me of this technique and having nothing to lose I tried it out with staggering results!

26. Move muscles into the position you want them.

Far too often I've gone for a back massage where I remain in the same position throughout the whole treatment and my muscles are never moved into another position. Moving the arms above the head, down the sides of the body and hanging over the couch, all change the way that you can access the muscles and get into those knots. Keeping the muscles in the same position limits how much access you can get to them and by adjusting their position you can work deeper into the muscles. This can be done for most muscles, such as bending the leg and working on the calves from the front, pointing the toes to work the achillies heel and bending the arm back slightly to work the chest. This is particularly beneficial when working on the neck and shoulders whereby getting a client to turn their head to the side whilst lying supine, means you can work the side of the neck more effectively.

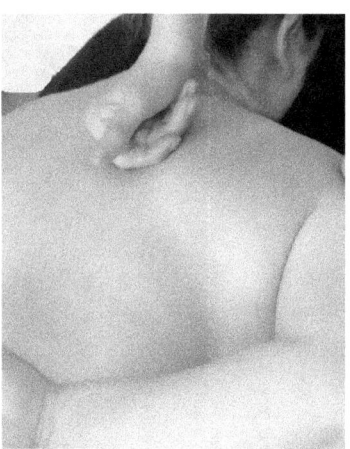

By placing the arm bent behind the back, you can work under the scapula and really help to loosen up the shoulders. By changing the position it means you can access the scapula and rhomboids more effectively. The feedback from clients has been very positive and they praise how they found the techniques very effective at getting into the neck and shoulders.

27. Not all massage has to be done lying down.

Typically massage is carried out on the couch with exception to treatments such as head massage, however massage does not have to be carried out purely lying down. There are obvious positions such as side lying for pregnant women in order to make them more comfortable. Alternatively massage can also be carried out in a sitting position. By carrying out the massage whilst seated it places the muscles into a different position and gives you an opportunity to work clients from a different angle. The seated position can be an effective way of working on the shoulders and neck and to carry out soft tissue work on these areas.

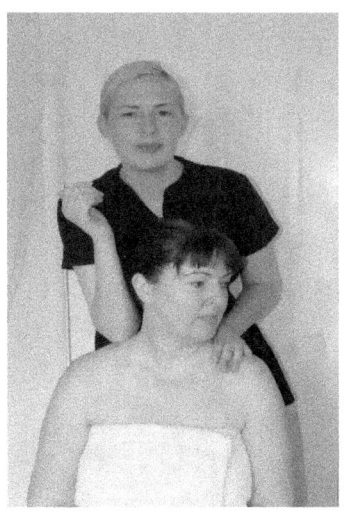

The seated sitting position allows the shoulders to drop down and places them in a more neutral position. Seated work provides a different way of working from the usual standard methods.

28. Release the shoulders by releasing the chest.

Often, you go for a standard massage at a salon and explain that you have tension in your shoulders and they get straight on with working your shoulders without any consideration to the chest. The problem though, is that in order to release the shoulders you need to release the chest. Thinking of the push and pull method; if the chest is tight thanks to all those hours sat driving, sat at computers, folding arms in front of us or picking up children, the chest muscles can become tightened and shortened. This can result in pulling the shoulder muscles around to the front creating shoulders that curve around. The knock on effect also results in lengthened muscles in the back and shoulders.

The muscles are then in the incorrect position due to lengthened and shortened muscles which can put extra tension on other muscles, such as the neck and can cause a build up of tension in the shoulders. Therefore you need to work on loosening the chest in order release those shortened muscles so they can move freely back to their correct position and put less stress on the body. Freeing the chest allows you to free up the shoulders and increase freedom in these areas.

29. Deep doesn't have to be fast.

Sometimes, the opinion is that deep muscular work has to be fast and relaxing massage is slow and flowing. However this is a misconception, in order to do go deep into the muscle you need to work slowly into it after having warmed up the muscle; the warming of the muscles can be quicker and more vigorous in order to get the blood flowing. Once the muscles are warm then the deep work can begin, which involves sinking into the muscles using a slow and deep pressure. Equally deep work is not about inflicting as much pain as possible on the client because a) they won't come back and b) it's not necessary!

Deep is not about painful uncomfortable pressure it can be gentle yet deep. Using too much pressure can cause the muscle to go into 'protection mode' and stay tight, due to excessive pressure beyond a client's comfort level. So remember deep is about slower work, sinking and working into the restrictions of the muscles, working to ease the tension out using varied pressure that does not have the client jumping off the table!

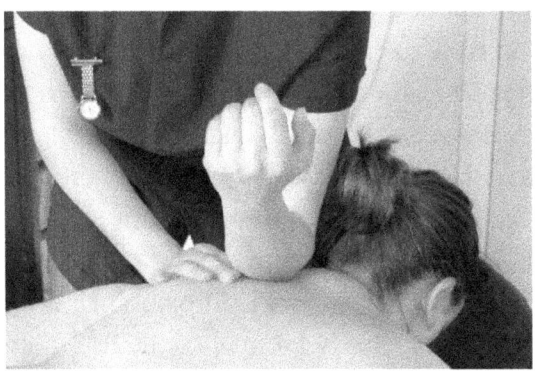

30. Golf ball technique!

A very well known but incredibly useful and effective technique is the golf ball trigger release. It usually involves placing a golf ball in a long sock, then throwing the sock over the shoulder so the golf ball is placed around the scapula or other key areas depending on what areas need working. The client leans against a wall and begins to move around so that the golf ball moves and works into any scar tissue or tight restrictions in the muscles, helping to break down those areas of tension and release any trigger areas. This technique is not just restricted to the shoulders, but can be used on the chest, legs and in particular on the lower back.

This can be a very effective technique for clients to use in-between appointments in order to continue working on their problem areas and get quicker results. Massage isn't about keeping a client as long as possible, it's about trying to help people get to the quickest resolution and this technique can encourage clients to do some self care in between appointments.

This technique is best done with a golf ball so it gets into those small specific areas of tension similar to how the knuckles are used. Alternatively and for less pressure, a tennis ball can be used, again placed in the sock and thrown over the shoulder and then worked into the shoulder, back and problem areas. The benefits come as a result of the pressure created by leaning against the wall and then gentle movement so that the ball can work into the trigger points and break down restrictions. The sock is used to help a client hold onto the ball a little longer, as without it the first few times can feel a little tricky and your more inclined to drop the ball!

FIRST STEPS TO SETTING UP

Think about what it is that you want from the business and visualise how you see your business being run.

31. Full time or part time?

When contemplating embarking upon a massage career you need to consider what hours you are willing to work. Whether you wish to work full time or part time hours. You need to look at the possibility that even if you wish to work full time, it may not be practical in the beginning due to bills needing paying and other financial commitments. It could be that you need to work part time until you've built up a sufficient client base to be able to work full time. Equally you may wish to only work part time as you enjoy another job and want to do massage on a smaller scale.

Depending on which option you go for you need to look at how you can pay your bills, taking into consideration that it takes around three years to fully establish a business.* You need to think about what hours you want to work and whether this will fit around your family. It is better to get the hours sorted out in the beginning rather than trying to change them later on.

* *www2.open.ac.uk/students/careers/exploring-your-career-options/self-employment*

32. Hours you want to work.

When creating your business you need to consider how you would like your day to look and the kind of times you want to work. So many times I've read on forums and equally I've made the mistake myself, whereby we were all happy to work whatever hours our clients wanted us to. If that meant we were seeing one person a day spread over six days, that was fine because we wanted our business to succeed. Who needs a Sunday off and what matters if your working every evening, the business is up and running, right? No!

It may seem simple and ideal just to work when your clients want you to, but resentment can equally creep in when you find your always working evenings or never have a weekend or Sunday off. That's why in the beginning it's a good idea to visualise how you imagine your ideal business to look, including the hours you want to work. Do you see yourself working three or four days a week? All day long or finishing at 5pm? Working certain evenings, working weekends? Think about what works for you, what hours you ideally want to work, otherwise before you know it your working five evenings a week, with daytimes free and clients only from 2pm or 3pm onwards, take my word for it it happened to me!

One way to help you decide your ideal hours, is to create a timetable with a column for each day of the week and then a row for time slots such as 9am – 12pm, 12pm – 5pm, 5pm to 9pm. Next, take into account your own commitments and what hours you want to work, filling it all in so you can visually see what the week could look like and see how happy you are with it.

33. Creating the right boundaries for you.

It's easy when starting out to want to bend over backwards for clients. To move your own events or activities or work that extra day even though you'd planned it off, just because you either don't like to say no or you want to accommodate all your clients. Once again, over time resentment can build up if you put your working situation before your own needs or that of your home and family. As the saying goes, take care of yourself so you can take care of others. You can do this by creating boundaries, including once you have created your ideal working hours you stick to them! So if a client asks for a Sunday and you don't work Sundays due to it being family time, you are able to say no.

When informing a client I'm unable to accommodate their appointment request, I apologise and explain I'm unavailable and then inform them of my other availability, that way there may be another slot they can make use of. This way you are not just saying no, but are giving them options and yet also remaining in control of your business! It's about saying no when things don't suit you, that you keep your boundaries in place. Therefore if you only work Monday to Friday you stick to that, if you don't work evenings you stick to that! However as we all know, saying no is never easy!

34. Working life designed around you.

Saying no is certainly not easy, but if we don't learn to say no and keep control of our business and work in our preferred way then resentment can grow. Feelings of annoyance and despair can occur because your not getting the time off needed and you are not in control of what you had wanted to create. For example, I don't work Sundays, I see this as a day for me and my life and I set boundaries in place whereby I turn clients down if they ask for this day. I display it on my advertising material and website so it's clear to everyone and I also keep my phone turned off and don't answer emails. Some people may be happy to keep their phone on and communication open, however for me it's about setting boundaries I am happy with and that means having a total day away from work.

By sticking with the days and hours you want to work, you stay happy knowing you are in control of your business. At the end of the day this is your business and you can choose the way you want to work. Yes there will be people that won't be happy because your unavailable when they want you to, but there are many others that will be happy.

35. What's available?

By telling clients what appointments you have available rather than them telling you when they want to come, they can decide from your availability and you will often find that it results in both parties being happy. It seems when people have less choice it helps them to narrow down when they can come, so that they can fit into the availability. I've often said to clients I can do anytime on the Thursday or Friday and then they stand there unable to make up their minds because I have given them too much choice!

Now that my practice is very busy, I will say ' I have Thursday at 10am or 2pm' and clients can decide from there. When you tell clients of your limited availability, this can also create an air of you being very busy. This usually implies you are popular and good at what you do and can encourage clients to try and find time to fit in with your schedule and value you further. I have had clients move things around because I only had Friday at 4pm available and they wanted that slot!

36. Diary, diary, diary!

The diary is king when it comes to running your business! Without the diary you have no idea where you are going to be and the busier you get the more you need to have everything in a systematic order! Whether you keep an online diary, paper diary, or ideally both, keep a diary of some sort and have it to hand at appointments ready to take the next booking. Having a paper diary backed up with an online version or vice versus is probably best as I have often had messages from clients informing me that their phone or computer has somehow wiped their diary and they can't remember when they've booked in for! So it's always good to back appointments up one way or another rather than just relying purely on electronic means! A page a day diary such as the academic a5 diaries are ideal as there is plenty of space to write down the time slots on each page and some even have times on the page. Remember the diary is King!

37. Men, women everyone!

When creating your business you need to think about who you want as your client. Are you happy and willing to see men and women or would you prefer to see one gender and not the other. This is your business and you get to decide who you would like to see as clients. Some women feel uncomfortable working on men, especially as sadly there are still some connotations surrounding massage and peoples perceptions of it.

The problem with cancelling out one gender means you exclude 50% of your potential clients. However if you market your business effectively, these issues can be overcome and you can see the kind of clients you want to work with. Firstly though you need to decide who you are going to work on, men, women or everyone! Only you can decide who you want as your client.

38. Mobile or practice?

When deciding on running a massage business you need to consider how you want to work. Do you want to hire a room at a practice where there are other therapists? Do you want to use a room in your home or would you prefer to run a mobile business visiting people in their own homes? All are viable means of running a business and you need to decide what option works best for you. Some people may hate the idea of being mobile and repeatedly carrying a table in and out of peoples homes, whilst for others it may be the only feasible option. One idea is to consider which options you prefer most and then create a pros and cons list to help evaluate which means of working will suit you best.

It's also worth looking at what other therapists in your area are offering to see what their doing and what appears to be working. Equally though, you may be able to spot a gap in the market and find for example, that there are a lack of mobile therapists in your area and this may work in your favour. Also make sure to check out your local area and see if there are enough people within close proximity so that you don't have to travel for miles or that there are enough people to sustain a mobile business.

You need to look at your local area and decide what works best for that, whether it's more beneficial to be mobile or have a base. If you have a town centre with lots of passing trade it may work better for you if you have a base, but if there is no particular town centre or lack of parking this may be problematic. You may prefer to work in a practice where there are other therapists so that you are placed in a less vulnerable position than working on your own.

However you have to way up the expenses of renting a room and the overheads, especially when first starting out as you may be making a loss rather than a profit and need to consider whether you have the finances to do this.

NEXT STEPS TO SETTING UP

Put the effort into your business, setting goals to support your businesses growth.

39. Have a plan in mind.

Business plans may seem as if there suited to a bigger business, but they are ideal for all businesses. If you don't know where you want your business to progress to, then how can you create the steps for you to get there. A business plan helps you decide how you would like your business to develop and what your final goal is. You may wish to eventually have a huge salon with various therapists working there or you may aim to see ten clients a week.

"If you don't know where you are going, you will probably end up somewhere else."

Lawrence J. Peter

Business plans can be downloaded from various sources online, indeed you can quickly and easily get working on your plan and begin setting it in motion. On a business plan there are various sections to help you identify your strengths, weaknesses and what resources are available to help you get to where you want to be. You may feel a plan isn't necessary or your plan may be only a loose version written on the back of a napkin, however you do it, it all helps to give you perspective and focus.

40. Setting work goals.

When starting out it can be hard to know how to begin or where you want your massage business to head. This is where the business plan and goal setting comes in. Once you've established where you want to get to you can work on creating the goals needed to get there. You can split these into short term and long term goals. For example, you may decide to begin with trying to see three clients a week. Alongside this you may set yourself the goal of only working one weekend a month due to 'family time'.

Now that you know you want to see three clients a week, you contemplate how your going to get there. You may choose to begin by setting yourself a goal of creating your website, having it up and running and giving yourself two months to do so. You may decide that in order to get to three clients you'll use Google adwords once your website is created or run a short offer to encourage clients to book.

Setting work goals allows you to break down your main goals into manageable bite size chunks and then turn your dreams into reality.

"Goals are dreams with deadlines."

Diana Scharf Hunt

Instead of worrying how your going to get to where you want to be, it gives you time to reflect on what steps you need to take to get there. You may decide that you would like to work more daytime hours. The daytime work is your main plan, so now you need to look at what goals to set in order to get there. For example, you may decide that you will run an offer for clients who book in before 12pm. You may look at what groups of people you can attract and who would book a morning appointment. Once you have decided on your target group, such as mums at home, shift workers or the retired, you can now decide to market towards that group by advertising in places they may frequent. Setting work goals means you can take ideas from your business plan and form a course of action in order to create the business success you desire.

41. Time, time, time!

One thing to consider when setting up your business, is that it really does take time to set up a business. It can take years to set up a full time self employed business and unfortunately success does not happen overnight or certainly only for the fortunate few! So instead of berating yourself as to how long it's taking and the fact the phone is quiet or no one seems interested in your services, realise that all therapists have experienced this at some point. We all sat there in desperation wondering whether it was worth it and whether anyone would ever want to use our services. However after perseverance and hard work to get your name out there, one day you get to turn around and see how far you've come and how full your diary is.

It may seem a long way off now but by setting your business goals, working on your marketing plan and website and creating a good online presence, you are setting the foundations to build a successful business practice upon. Even experienced therapists have weeks where they wonder why the phone isn't ringing or why their suddenly having a quiet week. Perhaps that's what makes us all good at our businesses, because we are constantly striving to improve our business. Keep in mind that it takes time to build a business and that you will have quiet periods and need to factor this in when setting up.

If it takes time to build a business how are you going to financially plan for this? Will you work part time and run your business part time? Do you have savings you are going to use? You need to factor in that your going to be earning less money in the beginning, so how will you meet this issue? These will all have no doubt been covered under your business plan! Mainly though, don't lose heart and realise that those first few years can be tough. However I can't emphasise enough the importance of putting the work in instead of expecting it to come to you and before you know it you can enjoy what your hard work has created.

42. Accept some quiet time.

Some weeks will be quiet and some weeks will have you chomping on your nails and wondering why no one is booking in! In the world of the self employed you need to accept that there will be some quiet times and not every week will be packed full of clients. You could sit there stressing about it and worrying how you will keep the business going or you could get proactive; realise this is a stage that happens and enjoy the quiet time or use it as a time to work on your business ideas. Running a business is all about taking it from strength to strength and in order to do this you need to have time to work on those foundations and that's where quiet weeks can be useful!

If you spend all that time stressing about work being quiet, when it is busy you will have wished you had enjoyed those quiet moments, at least during that time you could have enjoyed nature, caught up with friends and family, had some 'me' time or some business time. Indeed next time your having a quiet spell, realise that this slow period will pass and use it to your advantage turning it into a positive rather than a negative. An example from my own practice being, that occasionally I have some weeks where I have eighteen clients booked in and then the next week twenty five. I've gone through the motions of worrying when work is quiet and then decided one day to use it to my advantage and catch up on all those things I had been meaning to do. Even better when it is summer and you can get outdoors!

43. Knowing when not to take on too much.

Although there are those quiet weeks, the opposite can happen and there are those periods where suddenly you are no longer busy for just a few weeks coping with excessive demand but that you have been ridiculously busy for months. Whilst being busy is obviously wonderful and a dream of many business owners, what happens when you exceed that, when you get to that stage of almost resenting your business and the demands on your time and life. Those occasions where it has become the norm to work six or even seven day weeks, when finishing at 9pm is usual after starting at 8am. Those are the times when being busy is no longer fun but a draining chore and many of us get into this business because we love the work we do.

"Choose a job you love, and you will never have to work a day in your life."

Confucius

These are the times when we need to realise when is 'too much' and when it's OK to step back and rein in the control again. As therapists we want a thriving practice, but not at the expense of our own happiness. Often therapists talk to me about feeling guilty because their no longer happy with being too busy and that's just it, your not busy, you are 'too busy'. There is a difference. Being busy can keep us motivated and happy, being too busy makes us feel out of control and can effect the way we work as we end up spreading ourselves too thinly. You need to work out what is too much for you. Did you set out planning to work only two evenings a week and it's creeped up to five? If so, your already aware of what made you happy in the first place i.e. two evenings, you can then begin working towards cutting back and creating the kind of diary you want.

It's good to check in with yourself and find out whether you are taking on too much. People have commented that they know they've taken on too much when they become irritable, teary and feel they are swamped with pressures and no longer want to answer the phone. Put yourself back in control and get to a level of business that you are happy with.

44. When to say no.

Contrary to popular belief, being self employed doesn't mean you have to be constantly on call or that you cant say no when it involves extra work. Being busy is great but when it impacts on all areas of your life and when you feel your struggling to juggle everything, then it makes you aware that saying no is OK, at any time. Saying no isn't just about deciding to cut down, you may say no because you don't want to work that day or hours or have your own plans. Saying no isn't something you should feel guilty about, instead it's about realising the need for boundaries and the importance of your own time. Work is important, but family and friends more so and no one wants to neglect the needs of those we love.

"No matter how busy you are, or how busy you think you are, the work will always be there tomorrow, but your friends might not be."

Anonymous

Saying no can be very difficult though, especially as massage is a caring profession and you don't want to let people down. Practice saying it out loud to yourself or in the mirror so that you feel more comfortable saying it and it can make it feel less daunting. Saying no becomes less daunting the more you say it, just keep practising it and using it when you need it. No does become easier when you know what you are and what your not willing to accept. For example, I don't work Sundays unless there are special circumstances that suit me. I do not feel bad saying no to people about this because I've set my boundaries with regards to Sundays and know for me, working Sundays is not acceptable. By knowing what my boundaries and cut off points are I know when I am happy to say yes or no.

Saying no helps you keep your business running the way you want it to and prevents resentment building up. Practice saying no and if it is difficult then try with little things, such as not being able to change an appointment slightly and work your way up from this. If you would find saying no easier if you explained the reasons, then do so. That approach may not be for everyone as some therapists feel it's not necessary for others to know, however if it means the difference between you saying yes or no, then say no and explain that you have plans. It is clear, precise and honest communication which is always valued.

45. Not always on call.

It's easy in this day and age for people to constantly be able to connect with us and people often expect you to be on call 24/7, however this is not the case. You may be someone who is happy responding to clients at any time and if that's how you want to work that's completely fine. However, having talked to many self employed people the one thing they enjoy about going away is not being on call!

I tend to be on call when I want to be and when my hours are over for the day or it's my day off then I turn my work phone off and allow the voice mail to pick up the calls. This tends to help when someone chooses to call on a Sunday or at 7am and I have had all those calls before! You may choose to have a different work and personal phone so that you keep them separate and the work phone can go off when it becomes your time. Again this helps to establish boundaries between work and home.

46. Don't forget the tax man!

Benjamin Franklin said there are two things certain in life, death and taxes! So there is no point burying your head in the sand pretending that the tax man will magically disappear, he won't and he will still be knocking on your door! Instead of having a big shock when January comes, a sensible idea would be to put money aside each week to save up for the dreaded tax bill. I tend to work out what 20% of the week's takings are and then each week I set the money aside in a high interest savings account. This means that by the end of the year I have the money needed for the irritating tax bill. Don't let it creep up on you, open that extra account and start putting that money in weekly.

47. Carry change!

It may seem obvious, but you would be amazed at how many therapists I have heard from who've forgotten to carry change with them. If your charging clients an amount that isn't rounded up or they want some change then it always helps to have change on you, as you appear more professional, not to mention that clients will be wanting their change! I tend to carry a couple of £10 notes and some £5 notes and various coins so that I can ensure I have enough change to give people. I can't imagine how embarrassing it would be not to mention annoying for the client that you can't give them their money back and it could make them weary of you.

IT'S YOUR BUSINESS

This is your business, your way of thinking and your creation, run it the way you want to.

48. This is your practice, your way of working.

It can feel intimidating when a client comes to see you after having seen various therapists or having had a favourite therapist, with them informing you of how much they had liked their previous therapist. It can leave you feeling under pressure and questioning your skills, however this is your practice, your business and your chosen way of massaging. You can choose to feel intimidated by this situation or use the opportunity to ask how the other therapist worked and follow on from what they have done and found previously, thereby building on from their knowledge. Equally you can also choose to realise that you are also knowledgeable about the body and have your own way of working which may or may not be similar to another therapist's.

The client is coming to see you and they may love to tell you about how wonderful their other therapist was, however your going to provide them with the best possible massage you can. You plan to meet their body needs in the way you know best and if it differs from someone else's that's fine, because this is your business and way of working. Don't allow yourself to feel intimidated or question your practices, all therapists work differently and bring something unique to the treatment. Remember to value your own skills and have confidence in your abilities, as often by the end of the treatment a client is informing you they wish they had come to see you sooner and are quickly rebooking!

49. It doesn't have to be regimented.

Just because someone books for a one hour massage doesn't mean they have to have a full body treatment, it doesn't have to be regimented. Often clients tell me that they dislike being told what they have to use their time for. Some clients prefer areas being left out or prefer an hour on the back but feel forced to have to follow the therapists regimented routine, having no choice over how the time is used. When you are running your own business, you get to make the decisions and decide how the treatment is carried out in conjunction with your client's wishes. It allows for flexibility and imagination and allows you to provide a more unique service than other therapist's, whom are forced to follow a repetitive routine. It means that you can work with the client to find out what they like massaging and how they want to use their time, after all that's what their paying for.

At the beginning of each treatment, I chat with the client and ask how they would like to use their time. I'm giving the choices to them so they feel valued and that they can have the treatment tailor made to their needs, so if they want to have the whole treatment time used for the back of the legs and their back then they can. If a client wants their back doing and a short head massage, then how wonderful does that treatment sound and your not forcing a client to have muscles massaged that they don't want to. A massage doesn't have to be regimented it should be about giving clients choices so they can have the kind of treatment they want. Allow clients to use the time the way that best suits their needs and it encourages them to come back again.

50. What would you like with your treatment time?

We now know that treatments don't have to be regimented and follow the same old routine, which gives plenty of scope for being creative. However, you will have clients come to you that do want a massage but don't know what they want working. Also clients do not posses the same level of knowledge as us, so there may be areas that are best worked that people are initially unaware of. This means that you as the expert need to come up with some ideas and to think about how you would like your treatment time spent if you were the one on the table!

Always put yourself in the client's shoes and massage as if they were you. That way you give the best possible treatment as you are thinking about what you would like, which is sure to provide a soothing and beneficial massage! For example a client may not know that they can have a mixture of some work on the back and the head and they need you to be the one to create this treatment for them and it does tend to be a popular one!

A client came to see me and said they wanted me to particularly work on their head and neck, as this was where they were experiencing problems. I had a chat with them and explained to them the importance of spending time working the shoulders as well, as it was my experience that tightness in the neck and head was due to tight shoulders. Also from personal experience, I had often enjoyed the loosening of my shoulders so my scalp and neck felt freer. At the end of the treatment the client thanked me for spending time on the shoulders because as the massage progressed they realised how tight their shoulders were and the scalp and neck were less problematic. Use your knowledge and passion for massage to help create treatments to meet clients needs, whether it be for relaxation or remedial issues.

51. Clients you no longer want to work with.

Unfortunately at some point in your massage career you are likely to come across some clients who do not fit into your business for various different reasons. They may be overly demanding and insist you free up appointments for them, they may cancel all the time at the last minute or constantly reschedule. They may be rude or they may make it difficult to work with them. For whatever reasons, some people are just not designed for our businesses and are better suited elsewhere, if only for your sanity! Do not feel that you have to work with all clients and you can refer clients on if you feel their having a negative effect upon yourself.

When you have a client that you no longer want to work with, then you need to decide how you are going to get the client to move on. Often a good way of doing this is to chat with the client either face to face or via email, informing them that you feel they would be better suited to another therapist as you no longer feel you are able to meet their needs. Then you can list various local therapists you are happy to recommend them to or encourage them to search for other therapists if you are not keen on sending them to anyone in particular.

Another way of passing up clients you no longer feel happy to work with, is by recommending they seek alternative treatment. This could be through physiotherapy or osteopathy which may be better suited to their problems. Again chatting or contacting them to suggest looking for alternative treatment that may be able to better meet their needs and then listing alternative therapies.

You don't have to give specific details for no longer wanting to work with them and it's not very professional to tell them exactly what you think of them if you don't particularly like them! Remember to stay professional at all times as you do not want bad publicity. It's best to keep it short and to the point and to clearly state that you are no longer able to meet their needs, that way there is no room for changing minds!

There have only been a few occasions I have had to inform clients that we will no longer be able to work together. When I have had to do this, my response has been; 'After some thought, I feel that I am unable to meet your massage needs and feel you would be better suited to another therapist who can offer you the kind of appointments that suit you and that can meet your needs better. Here are a list of other therapists who may be able to offer you the service you deserve.' It clearly states that the client would be best looking for another therapist but at the same time explaining that I am doing so because of the desire to have their needs met.

52. Remain firm!

When you inform clients that you feel the need for a parting of the ways, this is likely to get a response of some description! Often clients will try and find a way of resolving the issues and if you feel the issues can be resolved and that you can find a way to keep the client, then do so. For example, if you no longer want to work with the client because they fail to keep their appointments, you may be able to chat further with them and inform them that this is their last opportunity and should they not uphold turning up to their appointments then you will have to ask them to go elsewhere.

Sometimes negotiations can be made and situations resolved, however this may not be case for all clients. Usually, once I have taken the decision to inform a client that I can no longer meet their needs, then that's the decision to terminate the relationship over and despite asking for further opportunities, I prefer to remain firm and ask them to look for another therapist. In some ways this may seem harsh, but if I'm working with a demanding client who wants more than I am able to give or who constantly lets me down or makes me feel uncomfortable, then I would rather have the clients I enjoy working with as part of my business. Remember, at the end of the day it is your business and your choice who you see and when you see them.

53. Only work within your comfort zone.

We stay our best when we are working within our own areas of knowledge and though it can be good to challenge ourselves, we have to remember that we are working on someone's body and it's not really time to practice when someone is paying you! Equally you may feel intimidated or pressured into carrying out work that you do not feel comfortable doing and you have to remember that you are completely within your rights to stay working within your own comfort zone. We are all trained in various styles and techniques, some more experienced than others and so we have to work in a way that we feel comfortable and happy working upon someone's body.

You may have clients coming and asking you to carry out various massage techniques that you do not know or feel comfortable doing so due to lack of knowledge. This is where you can politely decline to carry out that section of the treatment and inform them that you will refer them on to someone else. If you prefer to do relaxing Swedish massage and you have a client who wants more remedial massage which you don't feel comfortable enough doing or have the skills, then it's time to refer on and know that you are happy working within your own limits, after all we all have our own limits, strengths and weaknesses.

54. Referring on is OK!

One of the hardest lessons can be knowing when to refer on, knowing when your work may not be enough for the client or that they need a different type of treatment. We all want to do the best for our clients' and provide them with the best possible treatment, hoping that we will be able to help with their body issues. However we have to accept that we don't have all the answers and we need to consider what's best for the client. Referring on does not make you a failure or incompetent at your job, in fact it makes you good at your job as you realise that your client needs more than what you can offer. Always remember that it is about putting the welfare of the client first and about what's best for them.

Knowing when it's time to refer on can be difficult to gage, especially as some conditions and tight areas can take some time to release depending on various factors, thereby putting a generic time frame on it all can be irrelevant. The way I personally handle referring on, is that if I have worked on a tight area for a couple of sessions and the muscles are just as tight as the first session and that despite me working on them throughout the session they are still very tight at the end as at the beginning, then this makes me wonder whether there is a skeletal issue going on. If I felt we were not making progress I would recommend my client visits the osteopath. However this is when I have felt they have received very little benefit and with experience it can become more apparent when you should be referring on.

If I'm working on a client who has come to me because they've had tight muscles for a long period; I have seen clients who have put up with their muscular issues for years, then I will give my treatment much longer to be effective and will work with the client to create a programme to get them back to fitness. I could work on them weekly for several months and if I then did not see results I would suggest perhaps combining the treatment with physio or osteopathic work. In these cases I often recommend clients have a combination of muscular and skeletal work, because if their problem has been around for a long time, then the skeletal structure is likely to need treatment anyway. Basically, I refer on when I feel my work is not giving them much benefit and the muscles are not releasing and the client is still in constant pain.

ONLINE MARKETING TIPS
AND TRICKS

*You can be the best therapist but if you can't market your business
and get your name out there no one will know just how good you are.*

55. Website website!

I've met many therapists over the years who've often wondered why their business is not doing so well. When I get talking to them about their means of advertising, they often mention not having a website! How anyone in this technological world can get their business off the ground without a website is beyond me! It's second nature to us all to turn to the internet when we want to find more information and this is often the case when wanting to find out about services as we can read more detailed information about businesses online.

How do you expect someone to find out about your business if you do not have an online presence. By failing to have an online presence you miss out on reaching large numbers of clients. Research carried out by Simplybusiness show that 97% of internet users search for local businesses online and nine out of ten people call or visit a business found via a local search.

http://www.simplybusiness.co.uk/knowledge/articles/2013/05/why-web-presence-is-important/

Your website is your shop window, your opportunity for others to see your business and encourage people to get in contact. Without a website how do you expect people to find you and know your there.

First things first, get your website off the ground. You can either do this yourself, there are many simple packages online that enables you to just type away or you can hire a company to do this for you. We all have our own preferences so your best doing a Google search and finding a company or package that works for you. Don't submit a website that is half finished or with spelling mistakes or broken links. Not only will Google's search engine not like this but you need to make this appeal to prospective clients and if you are submitting a half hearted and sloppy website, this isn't going to give the best impression of your business. Remember to include your contact details, otherwise you will never hear from anyone! Equally make sure your contact details are displayed clearly, no one wants to waste time looking for these details or clicking off your website because they can't find them!

56. Less waffle, straight to the point!

When creating your website, remember less is more! You want to get your message across but without overloading the reader and putting them off. You want there to be straight forward information without the waffle, so that it's quick and easy to read and not time consuming, otherwise they may get bored and look elsewhere.

Bullet points work well to create simplistic sentences that are easy to read and convey vital information. Remember to keep it short and sweet, provide information but do not waffle on for several pages about each treatment or about how you got in to massage. All that information is important, but can be completed in less words than you think.

57. Don't forget keywords.

When you have created your lovely website, with enticing visuals, have cut down on the waffle and made it easy to read and are ready to submit your website, stop and check you've got relevant key words in there! If you have a fantastic visual website but have failed to think about the keywords you've used in your website then it may not do so well in the search engines.

The keywords are what they say they are, keywords found in the content of your website that will come up in search engines. For example, Mobile massage service Yorkshire provides..... or aching muscles...back massage from Healing hands massage service...mobile massage Hampshire provides. These are just some examples of key words which can be used in your website to ensure that your website comes up well in search engines. These brief keywords should realistically identify and describe your site so that people can find your site more easily.

Keywords help your website rank higher in search engines as they contain key information to narrow down a prospective client's search. When creating your website remember to contain phrases that reflect your business and location. Keywords are important, however don't go the opposite way and fill your website full of keywords to the extent that it isn't very readable or appealing to the reader and doesn't make sense.

58. User friendly.

How many websites have we all clicked on where it is full of lots of annoying adverts or overloaded with information? After a few moments of looking, you get bored and overwhelmed with the over zealous information or difficult to navigate pages. Not being able to access everything in a user friendly way, you come off that website and go in search of an easier to navigate website. Pages that are overloaded with paid adverts or lots of clutter can be off putting to potential customers and cause them to leave your site rather than taking the time to explore it.

By keeping your site clutter free with relevant and easy to read information, prospective clients can find information more easily and stay on your site. Bullet points are helpful with this as they allow you to convey information in an easy to read and quick format without all the jargon. Clients do not want to spend time trawling through your site to find answers, they want it clearly displayed and accessible at all times, so give this to them.

Cut down on the waffle, keep paragraphs short and to the point and without long pages of information. Make it obvious how to navigate the site by having clear accessible tabs and remember to always have a tab to allow them to go back to the home page! It seems many people forget this one! Pictures are great for catching the eye, conveying your message and giving people a visual taster of what you do, just don't overload the pages with lots of them or it can be off putting.

Websites that look half finished can be off putting as they make your business look sloppy and unprofessional. As always, think about what you would like to see on a website. We often take for granted, easy to navigate, clear and precise websites, but when you have seen how badly some people have done theirs you realise how easy it is to get carried away or to not put the effort in!

59. Facebook.

Social media is now playing a big part in the role of businesses from small companies to large. It can be a fantastic way to promote yourself and adds another shop window to your business. Some people will even use Facebook purely to search for your business, this being the only means they've used to find your kind of service so if your not on Facebook you could be losing business.

I've had numerous clients who've found me through Facebook alone and having a relevant and up-to-date Facebook page makes them look at your content more and know that your business is still running. If you have a page but don't keep it updated it can confuse clients and make them unsure your still in business causing them to go searching elsewhere for someone who is more active with their page. Facebook can be used to tell potential clients about the services you offer, inform people about how to look after themselves and encourage people to book in.

60. Blog it!

It may be hard to believe as everyone seems to devote hours to it, but not everyone is on Facebook! Therefore your missing out on a chunk of the market if you only use a Facebook page to advertise your appointments or let clients learn further details about your business. Just as with the Facebook page, I inform clients each week of my availability and keep this updated. Again, similar to the Facebook page I post quirky and inspirational e-cards and articles that I think may be relevant to clients, this way your not just trying to sell them something, but trying to give a holistic approach where they can find out more about their body and how best to look after it. It's an opportunity to show prospective clients about the depth of your knowledge reassuring them that you know about various aspects of the body.

61. Google adwords.

Google adwords can be a great way of getting your business out there and at the top of the search engines. It's particularly useful when first setting up and not many people have heard of you or during slow periods, as Google will enable many people to see your advert and web link that wouldn't have previously done so.

Google adwords is a pay per click advertising means, it tends to be the highlighted boxes at the top of the Google search or the ones to the right hand side. You decide on what your visible advert should look like and then set a daily limit of how much money you would be willing to spend. It may not reach the maximum level each day as it all depends on what people search and then click on, but setting a maximum level means you are protected from extortionate costs if lots of people decide to click through. When people search Google, your advert will appear in the relevant searches at the top ensuring that you are targeting your specific audience.

I am personally a fan of Google adverts as they were a great way of getting my business off the ground and getting my name out there. These days I am too busy for Google adverts however at the time they were very useful in getting me further up the Google ranking and getting people clicking through to my website. I also tend to go back to them during quiet periods or if I have a new service I wish to promote.

We all tend to be quite lazy and stick to only the first few pages of Google, ideally that's where you want to be and if you are on the first page so much the better and this is where Google adwords helps. You don't have to set a large budget to do this. When I started out, my daily budget was £1.00 and I would put £20 in each month to cover this. You can have more than one advert if you want to promote particular treatments and the relevant one will come up in Google searches. In the early days it's all about helping people to find your business and learn more about you and Google adwords enables this.

62. Google places.

You may have seen Google places when you've done Google searches in the past, they serve as a great way of promoting your business, especially if you can be one of the top few for your particular field in your area. Google places work by coming up in search engines with a map of services that meet your search terms and show how close to your current location they are. Google places is great, as like adwords, were all quite lazy and will only search those first few pages and Google places comes up at the top of the first page, just below the Google adwords sponsored ads.

It's another way of promoting your business and increasing your website presence, as well as allowing people to find your exact location. It's another opportunity to promote your 'shop window' and get your message out to prospective clients. Google places allow you to put information on there with regards to your services including opening hours and your contact details. If a client is using a mobile then it allows them to directly phone the business, i.e. you! Google places is free, so an ideal opportunity to promote your business at no cost.

The tricky bit is to get your business within the first few massage services for your area. Google always like it when businesses update their website content and Google places is no exception, so try and keep your website up to date. Also, try and encourage other people to leave a review on your Google places page as this can bump up your ranking. Once you register with Google places and set up your page you can email clients with your link and encourage them to leave feedback, which can help encourage further business.

Try and put up a few relevant pictures on your Google places page, as this can be visually appealing to prospective clients and make the difference between them checking out your service and someone else. Always remember and consider what makes you click a link to one website and not to another.

63. Update, update, update!

Once you've created a website and have it up and running it's not an opportunity to just leave it to it and put your feet up knowing that job is ticked off. If you don't get round to checking your website until several months later, then this can impact on your Google ranking and before you know it all that hard work you put in was for nothing as you see yourself go from being on the first page to being on the fifth.

By updating your website once a month it remains fresh and up to date so that people know your website is still live. Google can see it is a reliable and current website and keeps it up there in the higher rankings which is where you want to be.

MORE MARKETING TIPS AND TRIPS

'The aim of marketing is to know and understand the customer so well the product or service fits him and sells itself.'

Peter Drucker

64. Advertising your appointments.

One of the most complimented business innovations that I brought in to my practice was the advertising of my availability for each week. At the end of each week I post on my Facebook page and blog what my remaining availability is for the following week in order that clients know what options they have and it saves repeated questions about remaining appointments. Clients have really appreciated this initiative, giving positive feedback and sending emails or phoning to request a slot based on what I have said is available.

It's led to slots getting filled more easily and an increase in new clients as this way clients can see what options they have. Once I put the post on Facebook and my blog each week, I make sure to keep it updated so it remains current and relevant. Equally clients have also said that by posting my availability each week on their Facebook news feeds, it reminds them to get a massage which is a positive boost to business!

65. The importance of marketing.

You are your best tool for marketing and you need to work on getting yourself out there, meeting the general public and begin talking about your passion, which is massage! You can be fantastic at massage, but if you can't put yourself out there and meet people and talk about what your doing then your limiting your success. Someone can be a poor massage therapist but excel at marketing. They may receive a high amount of business because their able to sell themselves well and focus on marketing, either in person or through the many methods discussed in this book.

Marketing is the difference between your business being frequented by a few people who have been lucky enough to stumble across you or a highly successful business that continues to see a large volume of clients. You want your appointments full and you can utilise yourself by chatting with everyone about what you do. When meeting a client, you want to come across as friendly and approachable so clients feels at ease with you. Again this is all a part of using you to sell your services, by showing clients how much you and your business can meet their needs. Remember to stay friendly, warm and approachable and talk about the benefits without the overkill.

Another way of utilising yourself and getting your business out there is through network groups. There are many websites that you can use to find about one off or regular networking groups that you can join to promote your business and work with others to help sell your business. Again, engaging with others and selling the benefits of your service, showing the warmth of you as an individual will make it easier for people to want to come to you and for them to recommend you. There are talks you can do at local business centres, network groups and women's groups where you can give demonstrations and talks, if this appeals to you.

Remember you are one of your greatest assets when it comes to marketing. Make yourself approachable, knowledgeable and current and prospective clients will approach you more.

66. Think about your marketing.

If you are not careful marketing can cost you a lot of money, therefore it's important to think about how you are going to market your business so you get yourself out there at the best possible cost. Many therapists including myself have wasted money trying out marketing ideas that have got us nowhere other than a lighter pocket! Leaflet drops tend to have very little effect, yet many of us do them and find we have spent hours delivering leaflets to receive no response. Equally, signing up for pamper evenings at local events where you volunteer your time and services result in plenty of time chatting with people but again very little return with regards to new clients.

At first it can feel exiting trying out new ways of advertising, until you come to the realisation that these methods are costing you money but giving you no extra clients. Instead of wasting your time on these methods that the rest of us have learnt the hard way from, you can cut those bits out and focus on methods that give you a greater return. No one has an endless marketing budget and you want to be spending it on the right methods, many of which are listed in the several following points.

You need to think about who you want to be reaching, who is your target audience and how do you think they would find your business? Would they do a Google search? Would they look in a local business directory catalogue? Think about the kind of treatments you offer, if your doing pregnancy massage how are you going to be targeting people; leaflets up on the hotel notice board, contacting local NCT classes, using contacts who are pregnant to hand out leaflets? Again, think about all the ways that you think people would use to find your business and also how you would go about finding someone who was offering your service.

A lot of gyms and clubs will already have their own therapist, but if you belong to a club, there is no harm in you promoting yourself that way. There may be clubs out there who are interested in having a therapist attached to them, so it could be worthwhile approaching them. There are many cheap ways of marketing your business, the internet is key these days and websites do not have to cost a lot, Facebook pages and blogs are free tools and yet effective ways of bringing in business. Don't waste your money where it isn't needed.

67. Business cards at the ready.

I've lost count of the places that I have been where someone has asked me for a business card. It's always good to carry them on you as you never know when you may be giving them out. I was once on a train home from an evening out, when a gentleman sat next to me, it turned out we were both getting off at the same stop and began chatting. When I told him what I did, he informed me he was new to the area and he and his wife had been looking for a massage therapist. I gave him one of my cards that I always carry on me and a few days later this client contacted me and began having treatments with me.

It goes to show the importance of always having your business cards with you even if your off on a night out or doing the grocery shopping, as you never know if there is an opportunity to be handing them out. You can always get a business card holder to carry them in so that they stay neat and presentable, a smart looking card makes a better impression than a tatty one!

68. Not being complacent.

It can be easy once you've managed to get your business off the ground and are enjoying a healthy diary full of clients, to become complacent and to presume you will stay busy. Becoming complacent and forgetting to regularly market your business means there is no tide over from the busy to quiet periods and you run the risk of slipping down the Google ranking and having less of a business presence.

You are never too busy to stop marketing your business. Failing to keep up a continued effort can result in less clients finding you and old ones forgetting about you, resulting in a lack of clients and business coming your way. When you lose the focus, before you know it you are back to being quiet and have to spend several weeks trying to get yourself up to that busy level again, which can have a yo-yo effect on your business. You have to start the whole marketing process again, trying to get your website back up the Google ranking and update it so it's content is relevant to prospective clients and that their able to find you.

In massage, people leave varying amounts of time between treatments from a week to six weeks or the odd occasion. As a result, you want to be regularly drawing in new clients to fill any gaps and keep your business at a constant level with a flowing stream of clients. By keeping your marketing up to date and putting your business out there you ensure a regular flow of clients, new and old. Even the busiest businesses continue to attract new and prospective clients and who knows, the more you keep up your marketing the bigger your business can grow and you could choose to expand if you desire.

69. Referrals.

Once a business is established and you have clients coming through the door, it's about utilising those clients to get further business, by running referral schemes. Now if a client enjoys your treatment then they are likely to be telling everyone! Although some clients forget to tell others, you can encourage them to do so by giving them extra leaflets or business cards to give to their friends.

If your are in the early stages of business then offering clients an incentive is an effective way to get more business. When I had just set up, I ran an offer whereby if one of my clients referred three clients to me then they could have a half price massage treatment. This meant that I was at least getting that client back for half a treatment and still introducing three new people to my business who may go on to potentially book in future treatments.

I gave my current client a card with three sections on it to cut out and give to their friends, so that their friend would get a 10% discount when they produced the card, thus encouraging them to book in. Referrals are like a snow ball effect, get clients to introduce new people to you and before you know it they are becoming regulars too and guess what, before you know it their also recommending people to you. The referral scheme just helps to speed business up a little! Although this scheme may have cost me a little in the short term, it meant news of my business spread and I was attracting new business.

An example of this is my client, we will call her client A. She began having regular treatments with me and recommended me to her friend client B, client B found the treatments lovely and recommended me to her sister and brother in law so clients C. Clients C began having regular massages with me and then told their friends about me and so we now have clients D! From Client A I have gained five regular clients and have other one off treatments from their friends too. The power of referrals!

70. Filling certain appointments.

Some appointments will always get filled faster than others, such as evenings and weekends, but what if you don't want to work all those evenings or weekends. How are you going to fill those daytime or morning slots? Some of my clients love morning slots and others find it strange to have a massage at that time, it all depends on what clients you attract to your business.

One way of filling those less desirable appointments is by offering some kind of incentive, you don't necessarily need to offer it for a long period. You could run an offer for a month whereby if they book and have a treatment before 12pm then they get a £5 discount off their treatment. By running the offer for a month, you should get people who take it up and some may actually like or prefer it and keep with those appointment times.

71. Discounts and Offers.

Discounts and offers can be helpful in many ways to get your business established and maintain a steady flow of clients. Some therapists offer an initial discount when starting out, such as £5 off for the month of May, a half price treatment or a loyalty scheme such as have five treatments get the sixth free. Discounts and offers can be useful, by encouraging clients to initially book in and then loyalty schemes help to lock in clients for a number of appointments, whereby hopefully they thoroughly enjoyed their treatments and want to continue their massages after.

They can also be used to shift more difficult appointments, such as running a special offer for appointments before 12pm. These are all ways of targeting your audience and encouraging them to try someone new and different. Ultimately, with the intention of reeling them in further once they have tried your lovely treatments and turning them into regulars.

In my own practice I run a regular loyalty scheme, this is a rolling offer whereby a client receives a half price treatment every sixth treatment as long as the treatments are all taken within a year. 95% of my diary is made up of regular clients, in part due to the loyalty scheme which makes them feel valued as a customer and enables me to stand out a little from the competition; alongside them enjoying the treatments. Discounts and offers are a personal choice and some therapists are not keen on them, however they can be a great incentive for prospective clients. They can work particularly well in the beginning when you are trying to get established and you can always phase them out as your business continues to expand.

72. Getting rid of appointments quick.

When those last minute cancellations come in or you have appointments that you want filling fast rather than twiddling your fingers at home; you can try getting rid of them quickly. One way other therapists have chosen to fill appointments quick, is to send out a mass text message to their clients offering a special deal if they book an appointment over the next two days.

This can work well at filling appointments fast and re-jog clients minds about booking in again with you, especially as some feel put off that it's been so long. Plus it means your not stuck with lots of free time when you would prefer to be working. Some therapists have been known to halve their prices if people snap up same day appointments. It may mean you take a big cut but at least appointments that you wouldn't initially have filled are taken and you have money in your pocket.

You may prefer not to offer treatments at discount prices as you don't want to under value your treatments and work for less. However, this can be an effective way of ensuring that some work is coming in to your business especially when you are quiet. If you do this only occasionally, then clients won't become dependent on this method of having a 'cheaper' massage.

CANCELLATIONS

Cancellations happen, accept this fact, deal with it and half the stress is gone!

73. People will cancel.

One of the most important facts to remember, is that people will cancel! It's nothing personal and yes it is annoying but how you react to it is up to you! We need to remember that in our personal lives we all have events or situations that crop up which cause us to have to change plans, equally some people leave sorting or rearranging things to the last minute and forget to consider their other appointments.

Some clients may be fantastic and give you plenty of notice and then you are guaranteed to get the ones who think nothing of giving you two hours notice, rest assured this has happened to me! One week I had seven people cancel on me and five people reschedule, of which there was a mixture of between a few hours notice and a couple of days. It can be quite disheartening when you have planned your week and have perhaps had to change your own plans or turned others away. It really is a case of taking the rough with the smooth though, knowing when to be firm and when to be flexible.

Cancellations do require some flexibility. If your going to get cross and very firm with clients whenever anyone cancels regardless of whether an emergency has come up, then you are likely to scare some clients away! Alternatively, if your too lenient about it and do not remain firm and fair on other occasions, people can take advantage of you. Being flexible with regular clients and letting the odd occasion slip and encouraging them to give as much notice as possible, means you remain assertive yet fair, whilst keeping clients happy as well.

The thing to remember, is that cancellations do and will happen, they are not ideal and can be frustrating, but they are all a part of running a business. Factor this in to your business and go with the flow and you will feel less annoyed!

74. To charge or not to charge!

At some point you need to make that difficult decision as to whether to charge someone for cancelling at short notice or to allow it to go. There are times, such as in sickness or family emergency when only the hard faced therapist would charge and then there are those occasions where someone cancels two hours before their appointment resulting in someone else missing out, not to mention that your now out of pocket by losing an appointment. This is where having pointed out and made clients aware that you have your cancellation policy, then it is at your discretion as to whether you charge. Most businesses usually have a 24hour cancellation policy so you would be well within your rights.

This has plagued many therapists over the years as to whether they should charge or not and one point to consider is how much clients value your time and you. If someone cancels you at a moments notice without considering the impact on you, especially when they wouldn't do that for the dentist or other important appointment, then why is it OK to do it to you? Appointments cancelled with more than 24hours notice isn't a problem and is one of those things, but when someone cancels within hours of their appointment and it is too late to give the appointment to someone else then it is time to consider charging.

For a long time I chose not to charge people. However after a spate of clients with some in particular feeling it was OK to cancel within an hour or two's notice, I felt I needed to clamp down on this as it was leaving me feeling resentful, not to mention the financial loss. I decided to charge half the session cost to cover the inconvenience. Since doing this I have stamped out the number of last minute cancellations and feel that my clients respect me more.

Charging clients for last minute cancellations could indeed cause you to lose clients, although one thing I would consider is that it's better to lose them than have clients who don't respect you. Clients who feel it is acceptable to cancel at extremely short notice and then get annoyed at having to pay a cancellation fee and refuse to are perhaps clients you can do without. Especially if it frees up your business to take on more considerate clients who respect your time and skills and rarely cancel.

I've found that on the occasions where I have charged clients they've been the ones either insisting on paying or have been more than willing to pay or have been accepting of the situation. I do not make a big habit out of charging clients as I try to come to some agreement with them over responsibility, but on the occasions I have, I have not lost clients.

75. No shows.

Whilst there are those people who will cancel at a moments notice, there are those clients who won't cancel, instead they give you the pleasure of waiting outside their house for them to turn up or sit waiting for them at your premises! No shows are similar to late cancellations, they do happen, hopefully rarely, but they can happen and this is where you have a choice. Do you charge someone for effectively wasting your time and taking that treatment time away from someone else who could have benefited or do you accept the situation.

This tends to depend on whether they are a regular client and in these cases, unless there has been a serious situation or reason not to attend then I tend to charge half of the session price. This way it's not too much for them and equally there is no resentment then between both parties. I do know of therapists who would charge the whole fee though, so it is up to you and whether you feel there is a genuine reason or you wish to be flexible or if their usually a very reliable client.

I've had a small number of clients who've not shown and have ignored my calls. Hearing from other therapists, this is more common when you are seeing people at a premises. In these cases, sometimes it can be taking the rough with the smooth. You can ask them for the money, you can point out there is a cancellation charge, but sometimes you have to realise that this is the way it is and you can't always get your money back for an unattended appointment. In these cases, therapists often put that person on their list of people not to work with.

76. Deposits.

Some therapists, especially when it comes to larger jobs prefer to take a deposit for the booking. This is in order to help ensure the treatment goes ahead and if a client cancels a big job at short notice then this way they can recoup some of their costs. Taking deposits could be done via Paypal payment, cheque or bank transfer. This way it can be taken over the phone or online so the client doesn't necessarily need to be present.

For smaller treatments such as an hour's massage, most therapists prefer not to take a deposit. They feel it can put clients off booking, as clients don't always want to faff around beforehand and you don't want to scare them off. However for larger jobs such as for several massages or pamper parties where the number of people can increase or decrease at the last minute, this can help people to remain committed.

You need to let the client know that it is a non refundable deposit and will be subtracted from the total cost of the treatment so the client know where they stand. Taking a deposit may not work for all therapists, but for those who carry out longer and combined packages it may be a way of reducing the impact of late cancellations.

77. Making clients realise the importance.

You want clients to understand why it's important not to cancel so that you benefit from less cancellations and business runs more smoothly. This is especially true when your busier and you can't actually fit them in again due to being fully booked. In my practice I work a lot of evenings, I can almost guarantee my evening clients will not cancel or only do so in extreme cases. They work their schedule around their appointment with me because they know that if they were to cancel it wouldn't be possible to book in another slot and they would just have to wait until their next regular date. My clients realise that I'm in demand and they value the importance of keeping their appointment with me.

The busier you get and less easy it becomes to fit clients in, the more it seems they realise that by changing their appointment they will be losing out and so they put their appointment with you first. I also like to explain to my clients particularly those who tend to cancel last minute, that when they do this their causing other people who could have made use of the slot, to miss out. I do not attempt to make them feel bad about it, just simply point out to them that if they could give as much notice as possible, as someone else who is in need of a treatment could be missing out if they do not give me plenty of notice.

I try to get clients to realise the importance of their treatment with my business, because at the end of the day they'd try to keep appointments with other health care professionals so why not us.

78. Pointing out the cancellation policy from the start.

When filling in the consultation form with the client, make sure to have a section at the bottom to ensure they know that there is a cancellation policy in place. This way they know from the start what's expected of them and that a cancellation policy is present and ideally needs adhering to.

Displaying the cancellation policy at your premises, in a location that is easily visible by the client should help make the client aware that a cancellation policy is enforceable. It lets clients know they are entering an agreement with you and the rules of that agreement. Many businesses usually recommend a twenty four hour cancellation policy or a cancellation charge may apply.

79. Text reminders.

One way of cutting down on no shows or last minute cancellations can be through sending text reminders. It's amazing how many people think they will remember a date and then forget it or don't write it down. By sending a text message the day before, this serves as a reminder for people so that they will actually attend their appointment and if they can no longer make it then at least they can free it up and you can offer it again to others.

Some clients have forgetful minds and texts can serve as a great reminder, ensuring you cut down on people cancelling on you or not being there. After a spate of people forgetting, I began texting them so that it would help them to remember. Since then I have cut down on last minute cancellations and in particular no shows. All it requires is a simple message informing them that they have an appointment booked in for the following day.

80. Rescheduling.

When clients cancel, you want to change that cancellation into a reschedule, so although you may have lost their business that day hopefully they can fill up future empty slots. By trying to get a client to reschedule you could end up turning a new client into a regular client, all because you were able to accommodate them and give them a taste of your massages so they could see what they may end up missing out on!

Getting a client to reschedule means you don't fully lose their business, you merely end up postponing it slightly. When a client emails or calls to cancel, this is a good opportunity to chat with them and accept their cancellation and see if they would like to book in for another slot. You will be surprised by how many clients hadn't considered rescheduling or thought it better to cancel rather than inconvenience you, until you offer this option. Many times I have had clients get in touch to cancel and when I have got back to them with alternatives they have jumped at them.

Next time you think of simply accepting a cancellation, go back to your client and see if they want to reschedule and give them several alternatives. That way it is up to them how they proceed, you have given them choices and at the same time have tried to keep your client.

81. Back up list.

As we have realised, cancellations do happen and if you can plan for it and accept this, then you can use it to your advantage by having a back up list. For example, if a client has asked for a slot and it's not available, you can ask them if they would like to go on a back up list, when an appointment gets cancelled then you will get in touch with them.

Some clients find it hard to plan, therefore if you put them on a back up list and text them if you get a cancellation the slot may work for them and you are no longer stuck with an appointment that would normally be too late to get rid of. Creating a list means that clients who may sometimes miss out are first in line to get a slot that they would ideally like and you have less free slots.

This is also where the Facebook page really helps! I have had cancellations occur and within five minutes of putting the slot on Facebook they have been snapped up. The benefits of social media is that people are often on these sites and you are immediately hitting your audience.

KEEPING SAFE

Whilst we want to develop positive rapport with clients, we always need to be aware that we can be in a vulnerable position and the need for keeping ourselves safe and protected at all times.

82. Inappropriate advances.

The vast majority of our clients will be lovely and courteous people, however during your practice you may come across some people who are rather inappropriate in their behaviour. Sadly, there are still some connotations that massage is a sexual service of some sort; although this seems to apply to most therapies. Other therapists such as reflexologists have told me that they have also received inappropriate calls from people wanting an extra kind of service!

However, we know what massage is and how it is a therapy for the muscles and the mind and not for anything sexual. It can be a bit disheartening and unnerving when you receive a call asking for extra services, but being firm and explaining this is a professional service is usually enough to suffice. If you are unsure of the client, explain exactly what is involved in the treatment so that they are fully aware of what to expect from the treatment too and you get no nasty surprises when you are there.

Sadly it will happen where people get in touch and ask you for a different kind of service. Fortunately they are fairly direct and usually ask you if you offer extras or ask you if they are 'fully covered in the massage'. It may feel uncomfortable but at least this can be done over the phone and is resolved quickly. If at any point during a conversation you feel uncomfortable with a client, you can always approach it as many other therapists have, by informing them you have no appointments for several weeks which can obviously put people off.

83. No go.

You do not have to accept any kind of inappropriate behaviour. Equally even if the behaviour doesn't seem inappropriate it just makes you feel awkward, you do not have to massage that person either, its all up to you and what feels OK to you. If your working with a client and they begin to display inappropriate behaviour and I'm sure you can gage what is unacceptable behaviour to you; then you can either ask them to stop and inform them you will not be finishing the treatment and would like them to leave or leave the room and ask them to get dressed. They will no doubt know when they have been out of order!

If you feel unsafe with them, you can explain that you are suddenly not well and need to get home. It may seem like a silly excuse but if your unsure of the situation you are in, it can be a good idea to leave as quickly as possible whilst trying to keep the situation as calm as possible. If you do a massage and it's left you feeling uncomfortable and not wanting to work with that client again, then you can decline the client when they contact you at a future date. Perhaps you might respond by saying you are too busy and not able to travel to them or fit them in or similar to what was covered in the letting clients go section; by informing them that you do not think you are a good fit for them and feel they would be better suited elsewhere.

If they come back to you and question this, I would not respond unless they came into my premises and if that occurred I would inform them firmly and politely that we were not a good fit and I would like them to find another therapist. In these situations it is not wise to get involved with backwards and forwards communication. You have stated that you are no longer willing to accept this client and you are remaining firm with this despite what they may say. Trust your gut instinct, if you feel uncomfortable with them you don't have to work with them, pure and simple.

84. Self defence class.

If you are concerned about potential inappropriate advances and keeping yourself safe and protected, especially if working solo or doing mobile work, one suggestion is to join a self defence class. Self defence classes can teach you the skills needed to protect yourself against inappropriate behaviour if anything was to go sour.

Although the moves would only be used during extreme circumstances, having the security and safety of knowing you can protect yourself can make you feel more confident and comfortable when working with others. Alternatively you may wish to learn a martial art on a long term basis, but a self defence class will give you the skills to protect yourself often in a single class; although hopefully you should never need it. Classes can be found by searching online for courses in your area. It's always wise to do what you can to protect yourself, especially when working with others.

85. Staying in contact at all times.

It may sound like a chore letting someone know where you are at all times when massaging or giving someone details of your client list for that day but personal safety is very important. No one hopes anything will ever happen to them, but keeping safe is better than dealing with the consequences.

Several mobile therapists I know throughout the business, inform a family member via text or phone before entering a clients house and send details of where they are and what time they are likely to finish. They will inform them by text when leaving again so that should they not get back to the family member, it can cause some concern which may be necessary.

Alternatively if you are working alone at home or in a room, you can also send a message before a client comes and after, to a designated family member or your home phone, so that there are always records of your whereabouts should the unthinkable happen.

86. Same day appointments.

A lot of therapists I have spoken to choose not to give same day appointments to male clients in order to try and cut down on clients who may be looking for a different kind of service. Although this may seem a bit extreme I've had clients phone me at 5pm in the evening, staying in a hotel and wanting a massage as soon as possible. Although they may not have wanted anything 'extra' I would rather ensure I was safe and protected and decline the treatment.

The view is, that if a male client is looking for something 'extra' they are likely to want it as soon as possible rather than scheduling in for a few days time. Thereby offering an appointment in a few days time can cut down on those people who are looking for something immediately and may be desiring another kind of service. It's not to say that every person who contacts you at extremely short notice will be after anything untoward but it is better to keep yourself protected rather than putting yourself in a vulnerable position.

87. Ways to protect yourself.

Either working mobile, using a room at home or working late in an empty hired location, you are in a vulnerable position and need to do your best to protect yourself against anything untoward. Although it is very rare that anything does occur it's best to do what you can to keep yourself safe.

If you feel uncomfortable working with male clients then you may decide to work with female clients only. This may limit the amount of people you can see but it's your choice who you work with and who you are comfortable with. Alternatively you could ask that male clients have a female present for the first appointment so you can get a feel for your male client and feel comfortable with them. Equally you can state you are only willing to see male clients who have been referred to you by another client, that way you know them by association and have someone to vouch for them.

I would like to point out though that the vast majority of clients, male and female are very decent and honest human beings purely after a massage. Bare in mind also, that it is not just male clients you need to be aware of. You can not be sure of the actions of any human being and so need to keep yourself safe and protected regardless of a person's gender.

During the massage it is a good idea to set up the table and position the client so that they are furthest away from the door. This way if something untoward does occur, you are closer to the door and able to get out quicker. Carrying your phone on your person, means when necessary and if needed you can make a quick call wherever you may be and get help quickly, instead of realising you may have had to make a quick exit and have no means of contacting help.

Another possibility is to carry a personal alarm which sets off a very loud noise when the cord is pulled. This can send enough of a shock to the perpetrator hopefully giving you time to get away quickly. These may sound extreme and most therapists will never have to experience this in their career and usually a simple explanation that what your client is doing is inappropriate and won't be tolerated will suffice. However it is safer to know your options now and be able to put safety means in place.

Fortunately most of us have a happy safe and enjoyable practice, full of clients who always have our best interests at heart and who treat us as friends. Enjoy the business you create.

WORKING WITH CLIENTS

Clients come in all sorts of shapes and sizes, with various needs and problems. Put yourself in their shoes from time to time to understand their needs better.

88. Handling clients emotional baggage.

When working with people you have to remember that they will come with all sorts of issues, from problems regarding their bodies to emotional problems over none related treatment issues. Clients have often remarked to me that seeing me is like going to the hairdressers and they can tell me anything and often do! This can be a little overwhelming in the beginning when someone may be freely willing to tell you their life story or current emotional issues. In one way it could be seen as a compliment as they feel comfortable enough with you to want to share their issues. However it can be hard to handle or unexpected, so bare in mind that clients will be coming with all sorts of issues or life experiences to share with you.

We all expect clients to turn up for their massage but we don't realise that they will be bringing their home life with them, this is completely fine and part of a shared therapeutic relationship. Just imagine how you would like someone to respond to and listen to you. Clients are not expecting you to have all the answers or even necessarily to respond, they just want someone who isn't involved to listen to them. Next time a client comes in and tells you about their terrible weekend or falling out with someone, remember it is all part of working with people. All that is required is for you to listen and be a supportive ear.

89. Short counselling course.

When clients have a lot of emotional issues which they bring to the treatment and prefer to share with you, it can be difficult to handle. Although you try to support them, it can be hard going especially when you don't know how to proceed. It can be easy to get caught up in a client's issues so much so that your taking it home with you. One way to try and support clients emotional baggage whilst trying not to take on their issues; so always keeping one foot on the river bank and grounded, is by doing a short counselling course.

This can give you the skills needed to handle issues clients bring to the treatment, whilst allowing you to learn about being non judgemental and the power of words which can be useful when dealing with chronic pain issues which we discuss later. It can teach you the skills to create boundaries so that your not taking clients baggage home with you and your able to keep personal and professional boundaries.

These courses are usually six to eight weeks long, one evening a week therefore they don't require a big commitment but their benefits at helping to deal with clients issues can be extensive. Clients will come with all sorts of issues from family troubles to serious illnesses and it can be hard to handle these, but through a counselling course you can learn the skills needed to respond to your clients in an empathic way and in a way that keeps you safe.

90. Protecting yourself from others energies.

As we will look at later, some pain in the body can be caused or contributed to by issues of the mind and a negative outlook on life. I've had a few clients over time who have had very negative attitudes. This has resulted in me regularly having to challenge their attitudes in order to help them move on and for them to realise that they were recovering and that their emotions could be impacting upon their muscles.

I had one client who each time I asked him how he was doing he would focus on what hadn't improved or was still problematic. I would then get him to back track and look at what had improved since the last session and highlight to him any areas that he hadn't mentioned and then he became aware that there had been improvements.

However, working with clients who come with a lot of emotional issues or negativity can be quite draining and wearing over time. There are various ways you can protect yourself from these energies. One way is by keeping your feet literally firmly on the ground, feeling the ground underneath you gives that feeling of being centred. Secondly, you can imagine a protective white shield all over your body covering you from head to toe so that no negative energies can penetrate it but positivity can enter. This is a widely used technique that is often used to deal with negative emotions and other peoples' energies.

Thirdly, you can focus on breathing in healing, calming and positive energies and expelling any negative or overwhelming energies created by clients emotional baggage. You can visualise it as a lovely light entering your system and a grey miserable fog cloud leaving you. These techniques are all a good way of protecting yourself from the draining effects of negativity. Keep looking after you because in order to help others you need to keep yourself safe.

91. To talk or not to talk?: Some clients just like to talk!

When we carry out our training we are led to believe that lots of clients like to be quiet during their massage and this is true to an extent but there are also lots of clients who prefer to talk! It can be difficult to gage during the massage whether you as the therapist should talk or not. One rule of thumb, is that it's OK to talk in response to a client but not wise to initiate the conversation, unless it relates to the treatment and you need to know something in order to continue your work.

If you keep initiating conversation when the client is being quiet, they might not enjoy the treatment as perhaps they'd prefer a quiet and tranquil environment to switch off and relax and are just being polite. If a client wants to talk the whole way through the treatment that's fine though and their choice. It may be that this is the way the client prefers to relax and if made to be quiet they would find it less relaxing.

When it comes to talking, go with the flow, if the client wishes to be quiet respect this, if they want to chat for the whole treatment then go with that. However, try not to initiate conversation unless you feel it's necessary and is part of the conversation your having. Quiet or chatty, it's up to them!

MAINTAINING CLIENTS

Clients pay us to provide the best possible service. If we want clients to keep coming back, we need to keep meeting their needs and provide them with a reason to keep using our business.

92. Making clients feel special and valued.

When you have your clientèle built up you need to maintain this and keep clients wanting to come back to your business. You want to make them feel valued and to build a professional relationship with them so that they want to keep coming back to you. If your just going to chuck them on the couch, do the massage and then shove them back out the door, this doesn't make clients feel valued or special, it makes them think you just want their money.

You can make clients feel special by allowing them to make conversation on the massage table if their a talker. Also by being warm and open when they come for their massage treatments. By remembering things they have told you, such as the fact that they are going on holiday or that they have been having a stressful time at work. When you remember details clients have told you it makes client feel valued because your showing interest in them and are remembering things about them.

You can make clients feel valued and special by providing a treatment specifically for them. For instance, if they ask for more time on their shoulders you spend more time there, if they like deep pressure on their back but lighter pressure elsewhere you remember these details. It makes clients feel that their getting the treatment they want, instead of a mediocre treatment and that your listening to what they want from their session with you. This all adds up to a recipe for getting clients to come back.

93. Friendly reminders to clients.

If you haven't seen some clients for a while and want to encourage them back or to think about their bodies, then a friendly text to see how they are doing can encourage them to get back into the habit of having massages. Especially as some clients comment on the fact that they had been meaning to get in touch but kept forgetting to and then felt it was too long to do anything about it.

Having sent a message to several clients just to see how their doing I have got numerous clients to get back on track with their appointments. This isn't purely to attract them back to the business, but it serves as a way of telling them how important they actually are. It demonstrates that you think of them on various levels not simply as a means of helping you pay your bills.

94. Making clients aware of appointments.

Letting clients know about spaces available that they may be interested in due to them previously preferring that slot or having been after an evening slot but been unable to get one, shows you are thinking of them. If they'd said they were interested in a slot and you have an idea that they have forgotten to get in touch, dropping them a message can jog their memory and shows that you were listening to what they had said and considering their needs.

Telling clients about slots that they like shows you are putting them first which makes them feel valued and want to continue having treatments with you. If you know a client likes a particular slot or had been thinking of booking in but hadn't finalised anything, get back to them with options and slots you know usually work well for them. It shows you are considering them and valuing their business and trying your best to accommodate them.

95. How to keep clients.

In order to help build rapport and keep clients coming back, you need to remain in contact with them. For example, if they get in touch make sure you get back to them within a twenty four hour period so that they feel you are interested in helping them. Make sure that you use clean and comfy towels, sheets or whatever you choose to cover them. Make sure they are soft too! I've had massages before where I'm lying on old scraggly, rough towels, it was not a pleasant experience!

Another important point, make sure your client is warm. In the past I've had several massages that have been in a cold room with no music to keep me company and it wasn't particularly enjoyable. Although the therapist was good at what she did, the lack of detail in ensuring my comfort needs were met by warm or soft towels, a warm room and lack of music put me off going back.

Think about what would make you go back for a treatment and then apply those examples to your work. Such as, a warm and pleasant manner to greet people, contacting people back, offering alternative appointments if you have nothing to suit someone and staying on time but not rushing someone the moment the massage treatment is finished so that they do not feel forced out of the door and under valued.

Ensuring there is a gap between appointments in order that the next person is not there ready to jump straight in their place makes clients feel they have your full attention. Clearing and tidying the room ready for the next person after your client has left and not whilst they are in the room and getting dressed! Both of these have happened to me and it left me feeling like i was one of a chain of people on a conveyor belt!

All these factors add up to providing your client with a treatment that makes them feel they are getting a treatment above and beyond anyone else's. All those little touches make them feel that you think of them and their needs rather than seeing it as just another client and purely a business transaction. All these ideas are ways that can make your business stand out from the competition and keep clients loyal to your business because they know you are loyal to their needs.

PAIN AND THE POWER OF WORDS

Never underestimate the power of pain on the body and its debilitating affects. It can chip away at your physical and emotional state so that your no longer just working on the body, but mind as well.

96. The draining effects of pain.

When you are feeling fit and well, you forget how draining and tiring pain is and how it can affect every area of your life. Some clients come for relaxation, but many come for various issues having put up with aching muscles, problematic backs and nerve issues and some have been living with pain for what seems like a life time.

When you've had those feelings for some time, it can wear away the person you are, so that you become your pain and your injury.* *http://lifeinpain.org/node/2151* Never underestimate how tiring the pain can become, how it chips away at someone and how desperate they are likely to be to get rid of it. If you want to empathise with your clients you need to appreciate how drained and frustrated they may be from living in pain. How much they want to get rid of that pain and are hoping that you can provide a part of that solution. By appreciating these important points, you can show compassion to your clients that you understand how their likely to feel and how debilitating this is.

It's important to remember this when dealing with some clients who may appear demanding or desperate to have you 'fix' the problem. They may come across as angry and demanding of you, putting a lot of pressure on you. Remember how pain feels though so that you don't end up resenting them when their very demanding because all they want to do is to make the pain go away.

97. Acting confident.

Part of the process of helping heal a client is about the confidence you exude with regards to your ability to help. Similar to the power of positive thinking, if a client believes you can help them then you can help them. When you act confident it instils in the client a sense of trust and belief that their issues can be overcome and that you can work together to resolve this, you exude a belief in your service and the way it can help clients, that people can't help but trust in you.*

* http://www.womenunlimitedworldwide.com

Pain is more than purely a physical issue, pain can be in the mind and can manifest itself into intense pain, worse than the original issue. It can cause negative emotions and feelings of depression especially when a person doesn't know what's wrong with them and a sense of loss due to chronic pain and feeling worn out.* Thereby working on the psyche to convince it you can help, slowly breaks away at those psychological issues so that you can begin to work on the physical issues.

*www.healthtalkonline.org/peoples-experiences/chronic-health-issues/chronic-pain

When you ooze confidence it makes clients feel they are on the right path. It helps to create positive thinking which in turns helps to break down some of those psychological pain barriers. Also, by relaxing the body and mind through massage it helps to distract away from the pain and improve a person's psychological well being.

'....massage helped them to relax and avoid muscular spasms, but they needed a therapist they could trust not to hurt them.'

*www.healthtalkonline.org/peoples-experiences/chronic-health-issues/chronic-pain

Therefore never underestimate the power of pain and where it manifests from. As a great tutor on a course once said, massaging the body is like massaging the brain! Remember that when you work on the muscles you are working on the neurones that go to the brain, so work the brain and the muscles together.

98. Believe in yourself.

When clients come to you desperately in pain or in need of some serious de-stressing, they are putting their faith and hope in you. They are trusting that you can help; if you don't believe in yourself how can you expect others to believe you can help them. You want to be instilling confidence in them and you can do this by believing you have the skills and knowledge to help your clients with their issues.

Clients can end up listening to every word you say and are happy to follow through your advice because they believe you know what your talking about. However if you come across as unsure or tell your clients that you don't know or your very hesitant, then this hardly instils confidence in them and can make them doubt your expertise. This in turn can result in them looking elsewhere for a therapist. They could end up looking for another therapist because they no longer believe in you, when actually you had the knowledge and skills all along but didn't feel confident in your own abilities. So next time you begin to doubt yourself, realise that your clients believe in you and the power of your work and that their listening to what you have to say. They have confidence and belief in you so need you to act that way.

If you don't feel overly confident in your abilities, then further study can help you to believe in your skills. Consider CPD courses that allow you to question and develop your skills. Self development work, such as reading massage books, magazines and articles by well known massage therapists such as Art Riggs and Erik Dalton, can all increase your knowledge and self belief.

99. Never underestimate pain in the mind.

Pain can manifest both as physical pain but it can also be a psychological pain that appears to be physical. We all hold traumas within our bodies, whether from a nasty break up, a bereavement or stresses at work. Over time they can add up and build upon one another, especially if we've been going through a difficult time over several months or years. We begin to take on that emotional trauma, holding it in our bodies and becoming accustomed to that feeling, to the extent that we don't feel we can cope without holding on to that trauma.*

* *http://www.cellularmemory.org/about/about_painbody.html*

When we massage the body, we can help to chip away at the psychological pain, hence informing clients they can feel heightened emotions after the treatment. We can do this through the techniques we use, such as massing the chest and shoulders to open up the body so the client feels stronger and less curled up in a protective pose, almost as if they are ready to receive the world. However, clients can be used to holding onto this trauma and using it as a coping mechanism and subconsciously may not be willing to give this up. We need to be aware of this when working with clients as this psychological pain could be a reason why clients are not seeing improvements and could be an area that needs working on for clients to move forward with their treatment.

By regularly massaging clients we encourage them to take better care of themselves and to slowly deal with any emotional issues that come up due to slowly releasing the tension. We can support out clients with their psychological pain by talking with clients about their physical issues and anything that comes up for them as and when they want to. By working the physical issues we can help support clients with their emotional issues. There are some clients that we can work on their physical problems but due to their emotional issues we are unable to fully help, however it is up to these people to take their own steps and we can support them with their physical needs.

100. Clients trust in you.

If a client has been in pain for some time, they are often desperate to get their issue sorted, as well as feeling despondent that nothing will work and worn down by feeling the way they have done. Therefore when you act confident it makes clients want to trust in you and believe you can help. It begins the process of getting their bodies back in shape as it can remove some of this negative energy they have been feeling as they begin to trust in you and believe that you can resolve some of their issues.

When a client trusts in us, we have to maintain that belief and we can do this through the words we use and by instilling positivity into the client. Just as you should never underestimate pain in the mind never underestimate how far the effect a client's trust and belief in you can go, in order for them to heal. By instilling confidence in your client so that they trust you, your able to break down some of those pain barrier issues and help with emotional issues such as the fear that no one can help them.

Clients will only trust in you if you come across as knowledgeable and are able to instil confidence in them that their issues can be resolved. If your going to stand in front of them umming and ahhing and seeming unsure, then they will not feel confident in you. Barriers can go up as they feel uncertain of your skills and ability to help them. Remember that what you say impacts upon the client, hence the need for positive language and explaining clearly to them what you are working on and your findings. Once you begin the massage and start breaking down the tension, the trust often begins to flow but requires being backed up by positive language and an understanding of their health.

101. Choose your words carefully.

When working with clients and especially those with issues, you need to think about the words you use in order to encourage them to get better and move away from negative attitudes. When a client has a negative attitude towards their health and body issues and are hung up on how their not doing so well, you want to work on changing that attitude and one way of doing this is through the words we use. By choosing your words carefully and using positive language you can encourage clients to change their attitudes and see that their health is in fact improving. By using choice words you can steer them away from seeing the downside of their situation and seeing what has improved.

For example, a client of mine when asked how he was each week would always start and end with how bad his body was. I would get him to check over what had actually improved or how long it was before he felt his muscles tighten up or would mention specific areas he had been complaining about previously. This prompted him to do another check of his body and realise that some things had improved and that he was making progress, which made him feel better about his health.

It's not to say that we shouldn't acknowledge negative feelings or pain issues, just that by choosing our words carefully we can encourage clients to see all aspects of their health. If you continue to agree with your client about how much pain their in or how bad their body issues are, then it allows this whole melancholy atmosphere and doesn't leave much room for improvement.

HOLISTIC APPROACH

When we massage people we are not just working on the body, we need to consider the whole person, from the muscles to the mind and all that's in between.

101.1 After care advice.

After care advice is an opportunity to let clients know how best they can look after themselves in between appointments and helps to give a holistic approach. It shows clients that you are thinking about them above and beyond just their massage treatment. It's an opportunity to inform clients of how best they can prolong the benefits of their massage treatment.

We all know the basic after care advice, i.e. drink lots of water, you may feel sleepy, avoid toxins and so forth. However, we are trying to show our clients that we are more than just an average massage business, we have their interests at heart and were committed to meeting their needs. Therefore you want after care advice that's exceptional and gives the client something they can work towards, including for those clients particularly in need, by creating a type of ongoing programme of after care advice.

After care advice that considers the whole person is one that focuses upon the use of exercise to help maintain good muscle strength and healthy muscles. It also encourages clients to look at their lifestyle, questioning whether they are stressed and need to incorporate more relaxation techniques such as hot baths, meditation, time out and listening to relaxing music to name but a few. If you advance your massage skills to remedial or sports, you may look at various exercises the client can do to help keep themselves looser for longer and help build up strength in weak muscles.

When giving advice to clients who have come due to perhaps aching muscles or problem areas, you want to make them aware that it can take time to break down muscle tension and is a gradual but beneficial process. It's important clients are made aware of this so that they realise it is a journey and do not have unrealistic expectations believing that their problem will disappear immediately. This way they are not disheartened when tension begins to come back. Remind them that the tension has been there for some time so it will take time to break down, but each session helps to chip away at it a bit more. Remind them that their muscles may hurt after the massage treatment, especially if they've had some deeper work done!

101.2 Begin to learn about exercise.

With all the advice in this book we are really beginning to show how exceptional and professional our business is and the holistic approach we are able to give with the client at the centre of it.   In order to continue that holistic approach and following on from the after care advice, we want to be looking at providing the client with relevant exercises that help with any muscular issues they may have.

Remember that as far as the client is concerned, you are the expert, they want and are likely to be relying on your advice to help meet their needs. Over the years I have been asked numerous weird and wonderful questions by clients, but exercise and the best exercises to do, is one that comes up repeatedly if I haven't already offered this first. Therefore it helps to begin to get to grips with exercise and the best exercises for releasing tension so you can advise your clients.

A simple internet search will be able to provide plenty of relevant information and give you a base for finding out more about the relationship between tension and muscles. Ideally you want to be looking at exercises that help to open up the chest and get the shoulders back. You want to include exercises that focus on strengthening core muscles which will in turn help the lower back. Further exercises include those that strengthen the shoulders, stretches to free up the lower back and stretch out the neck. You can go on to do more in depth stretching courses, providing you with greater knowledge of stretches that you can tailor for your client.

101.3 The holistic approach.

Remember that the after care advice you give is more than simply focusing upon the massage and the effects from it. There is always a focus upon the whole person and remembering that pain created in the mind can be a huge contributing factor therefore we can't just focus upon the physical issues or muscles.

Taking into account de-stressing techniques, exercise and diet, means we look at various factors that may be contributing to any issues. Even if a client has no specific issues, we always want to be looking at the whole person rather than giving them generic advice relating purely to the massage.

101.4 Learn your stuff, become the knowledgeable one.

What makes someone a good therapist and someone a great therapist? Someone who is passionate and knowledgeable about their subject, someone who makes the decision to become the knowledgeable one! I remember when I first became a massage therapist, I was reading an online forum and wondering what all these strange technical terms were. Fast forward several years and it's a wonderful feeling to know that the advice you are giving clients and your response to their issues is the same as what the osteopaths and physiotherapists are giving.

Becoming the knowledgeable one involves you making a decision to learn more about the body. To continue your professional development, to read up about muscles and exercise and to follow some of the gurus of massage depending on what your discipline is. When you chat with a client and are able to inform and point out to them areas of tension or trigger point techniques to release tight muscles on their own; your displaying to them that you are knowledgeable about your subject. Your demonstrating you can approach it from various angles in order that they get the best benefit. When a client sees your commitment to them in this way, it encourages and confirms their commitment in you.

101.5 Practice what you preach.

If you are going to stand there and tell clients that they should take care of their bodies, that they should have regular massages to sort out aches and pains and to maintain their bodies, then you should really be practising what you preach. What is the point in telling others to look after themselves if your unable to do the same yourself.

We want people to return to massage because we know how beneficial it is and how it can help look after us, so if we know this, shouldn't we be having regular massage ourselves? Practice what you preach! Follow through on that exercise routine because you know it helps strengthen your body and keeps you fitter and healthier for work. Have that regular massage because you know how good it makes you feel. That way, you can stand in front of clients knowing you truly believe in what you are practising and in the advice you are giving to others. You believe in the power of massage and are making sure you reap the benefits of this wonderful treatment, just as your clients do.

Pearls of wisdom

Realise a business takes time.

No one grows a business over night, although that really would be wonderful. Instead we have to slog away at it and put the hard work in and accept it takes time. Each occasion you find yourself getting frustrated at how slow everything is going, remember it will take as long as it takes and it always takes some time to develop a business. Remember this fact and it will save you some stress!

Realise that you don't have to say yes to everything.

Just like you don't say yes to every invitation, task or favour asked of you, the same applies to your business. You can't possibly say yes to every request, so get in to the habit of saying no early on in your business and you will feel less under pressure. Just because someone asks you doesn't mean you have to say yes, saying no is not a bad word! Remember that!

That by being firm and strong you show people you mean business.

We've all heard the phrase, give people an inch and they will take a mile. Remember to stay firm and stick to what suits you even if it means saying no to clients. By being strong and sticking to your boundaries you create a business that you want and one that clients have to respect.

The diary is King.

We can not live without our diaries, they hold our key information. Invest in one from the beginning and it will help ensure you never miss an appointment. Carry it with you wherever you go or have it always available ready for that next booking. Realise it is a key part of your business and never be without it!

Don't let people dictate your slots.

Only you get to decide your diary. You will get some clients who feel that from the moment they meet you that they can dictate exactly when they see you regardless of what your diary says. If you already have someone booked in then or do not work those days, don't let them dictate. Some people are used to getting exactly what they want and demand from people. Sometimes this isn't possible and they have to work with what you have no matter how intimidating they can be.

Keep clients warm.

No one likes being cold, especially when receiving a massage. You fail to keep your clients warm and it could be the reason they don't come back. Use a heated blanket on the couch, a warm blanket, a heated room, whatever nice touch you feel will help keep your clients warm.

Be good at what you do.

Try and be the best therapist you can be, put your heart into creating a business that you would want to go to. Don't forget to expand your skills and continue developing your knowledge so that you become great at what you do. Learning is a life long commitment, don't become complacent.

Takes hard work.

You are going to have to put in the hard work! You are going to have to work to draw clients to your business, to get your name out there, to make your business successful. During those times when you wonder 'what is the point' remember that everyone else had those same thoughts but they got there through hard work.

Put the hard work in and you will see your business grow and develop.

Turn off the phone.

Would you really want a massage where someone's phone is constantly ringing. Having experienced this, it is not pleasant or conducive to relaxation. Life can go on without you needing to be attached to your phone! Pop your phone on silent, that way it doesn't disturb the massage.

Enjoy it!

This is your adventure, your journey. Yes there will be some difficult times, some frustrating and worrying times, but there will also be some fantastic and rewarding times. Enjoy the journey! Enjoy the moment when you find yourself seeing ten clients a week, enjoy the feedback when you hear back from clients saying how much they have benefited from your treatment. Enjoy what you do.

There you have it, hopefully you now feel well informed and confident to grow your massage business, taking it from good to great.

There may be some bumps and steep hills, but enjoy the journey of your massage career. Enjoy creating the business you want and your adventures in helping others.

I wish you all the luck in the world....

ABOUT THE AUTHOR

Dannie has worked in the therapeutic industry as a massage therapist for over six years, developing the skills and knowledge required to run a busy massage practice. Struggling through the various different way of setting up a business and building a client base, learning the hard way that leaflet drops don't work and how to get clients to come back, she gained the knowledge to create this insightful book. Deciding to help others to cut out some of the hard work and lessons so they can develop their own thriving businesses.

When Dannie is not pummeling muscles she can be found on the other side of the couch indulging in massages! She enjoys experiencing life through her travels and keeping active through kayaking.